THE NEW MEDICAL SOCIOLOGY

SOCIAL FORMS OF HEALTH AND ILLNESS

Contemporary Societies Series

Jeffrey C. Alexander, Series Editor

Forthcoming

THE NEW MEDICAL SOCIOLOGY

Social Forms of Health and Illness

Bryan Turner
UNIVERSITY OF CAMBRIDGE

CONTEMPORARY SOCIETIES
Jeffrey C. Alexander
SERIES EDITOR

 W. W. NORTON & COMPANY ☉ NEW YORK LONDON

W. W. Norton & Company has been independent since its founding in 1923, when William Warder Norton and Mary D. Herter Norton first published lectures delivered at the People's Institute, the adult education division of New York City's Cooper Union. The Nortons soon expanded their program beyond the Institute, publishing books by celebrated academics from America and abroad. By mid-century, the two major pillars of Norton's publishing program—trade books and college texts—were firmly established. In the 1950s, the Norton family transferred control of the company to its employees, and today—with a staff of four hundred and a comparable number of trade, college, and professional titles published each year—W. W. Norton & Company stands as the largest and oldest publishing house owned wholly by its employees.

Manufacturing by Quebecor World—Fairfield Division.
Book design by Beth Tondreau Design, New York.
Production manager: Benjamin Reynolds.

Library of Congress Cataloging-in-Publication Data
Turner, Bryan.
    The new medical sociology : social forms of health and illness / Bryan Turner.
        p.   cm.— (Contemporary societies)
    Includes bibliographical references and index.

ISBN 0-393-97505-3 (pbk.)

    1. Social medicine.   I. Title.   II. Series.

RA418.T9115 2004
306.4'61—dc22

                                                                    2004043475

W. W. Norton & Company, Inc., 500 Fifth Avenue, New York, N.Y. 10110
www.wwnorton.com

W. W. Norton & Company Ltd., Castle House,
75/76 Wells Street, London W1T 3QT

1   2   3   4   5   6   7   8   9   0

To Eileen

CONTENTS

ACKNOWLEDGMENTS

THE ARGUMENTS AND CONTENTS of this volume are an original contribution to the development of medical sociology. Furthermore, the book aims to provide a coherent and integrated approach to the sociological study of health and illness that draws on the classical legacy of sociology. In developing this study, I have drawn on previously published ideas and arguments: B. S. Turner, "The History of the Changing Concepts of Health and Illness: Outline of a General Model of Illness Categories" (2000a); "Disability and the Sociology of the Body" (2001); B. S. Turner, "Risks, Rights, and Regulation: An Overview" (2001a); and B. S. Turner, "Social Capital, Inequality, and Health: The Durkheimian Revival" (2003a). I am grateful to Gary Albrecht for his support of my interest in the sociology of the body, for his encouraging me to apply these ideas to impairment and disability, and for his permission to use aspects of these chapters in this study. Professor Andrew Alaszewski helped me compose the original article on risk and has encouraged me to develop the argument in this textbook. Graham Scambler and Paul Higgs have kindly supported my interests in social theory in the field of medical sociology.

Both Mike Featherstone and Mike Hepworth have been important in the development of the sociology of the body and aging and have in many ways influenced the development of this study. Many of the ideas that have shaped this book have emerged from my editing *Body & Society* with Mike Feather-stone over the last decade. Darin Weinberg, with whom I teach medical sociology in the Social and Political Sciences tripos at Cambridge, has been enormously helpful in framing my criticism of social constructionism—a criticism with which he largely disagrees. Mary Evans was helpful specifically in encouraging me to abandon the idea of human frailty in favor of the more subtle and interesting notion of vulnerability—a key concept in this approach to health and illness.

For some years, it has been my privilege to serve as an advisory editor of *Social Science & Medicine*. The journal and the articles I evaluate have helped me establish the self-critical criteria of scholarly excellence in medical sociology to which I aspire, and they have been particularly important in developing this approach to social capital theory in health and illness. I owe particular thanks to Sally Macintyre and Mildred Blaxter for their continuing support and confidence in me.

I am also grateful to the following people for advice, support, and encouragement: Jeffrey Alexander, Jack Barbalet, Liz Chapman, Randall Collins, Oona Corrigan, Tom Cushman, Peter Dickens, Robert Dingwall, John Dunn, Gary Easthope, Dani Fleck, Arthur Frank, John Germov, Peter Hamilton, Paul Higgs, Engin Isin, Sue Kenny, Arthur Kleinman, Frank Lewins, Tony Manstead, John O'Neill, Martin Richards, Roland Robertson, Chris Rojek, Colin Samson, Graham Scambler, Wendy Seymour, Chris Shilling, Ken Thompson, Steven Wainwright, Kevin White, Simon Williams, and Evan Willis.

My colleagues at Cambridge have been wonderfully supportive, especially in recent years, through my own illness episodes: Geoff Ingham, Christel Lane, David Lane, David Lehmann, Jackie Scott, John Thompson, and Darin Weinberg. Brian Johnson, Master of Fitzwilliam College, has been characteristically enthusiastic about my projects. A host of students have patiently endured draft versions of the ideas that finally shaped this book.

Melea Seward and Stephen Dunn generously provided invaluable editorial assistance and greatly improved the original draft manuscript.

Intellectual stimulation and inspiration from the late Philip Strong, whose untimely death robbed British sociology of a creative and acute mind, originally ignited my interest in health and illness as core topics of sociology.

My sincere thanks go to the staff of Addenbrooke's Hospital, Cambridge, who kept me alive through the summer of 2001 and the spring of 2003, and to my fellow patients, who provided endless and poignant narratives of vulnerability, suffering, and courage. My final thanks go to my wife, Eileen Richardson, who cared for me throughout.

Fitzwilliam College, Cambridge, April 2004

INTRODUCTION

SOCIOLOGY IS THE SCIENTIFIC STUDY of social institutions. Institutions are clusters of social roles and norms that structure individual behavior and practice. Legal institutions are particularly important in shaping our behavior, by compelling us, if necessary by force, to obey certain regulations. Institutions are receptacles of power and knowledge. They determine how we see, experience, and understand social reality. Medicine, like religion, is a social institution, a collection of social roles, practices, associations, codes, and systems of knowledge that shape the direction and characteristics of modern society. If a person develops a serious or traumatic condition, such as pancreatitis, his or her experience of the acute condition and the medical response to the problem produce a major disruption in the social routines of everyday life and may well bring about significant changes in self-definition. The sociological study of health and illness not only addresses such subjective experiences of acute and chronic conditions in our daily lives but also considers important economic and political issues that ultimately determine disease and sickness. Sociologists study the interface between institutions and experiences. The sociological imagination makes the historical and social connections between our personal troubles and larger issues in the social structure (Mills 1959). Medical sociology studies the personal narratives of our health troubles but understands them in the context of large-scale economic, political, and social processes.

The field of medical sociology is important not only because health is increasingly a measure of the good society but also because it plays a part in social control and thus raises political issues about social and human rights (Zola 1972). When we voluntarily follow a physician's advice about how to manage something that is troubling us, we accept a medical regime. The word *regime* should remind us of related ideas, such as regiment or regimentation. In accepting a medical regime, we undertake to control our lives in various ways, through diet, exercise, or more generally, lifestyle. The word *diet* is connected to the term *government*, and hence when we follow a doctor's orders, we impose a government on our lives. Medicine regulates our lives through a contract that we implicitly make with the doctor. Through such everyday processes, medical science plays a significant part in defining what is regarded in society as normal. What is healthy is now what is normal. In sociology, the social processes whereby social activities come under the control of medical institutions are called medicalization in order to indicate the power of medical institutions. More precisely, medicalization involves the use of medical explanations and modes of medical thinking across different areas of society, for example by explaining criminal behavior as a consequence of a medical condition (Conrad 1992). People who are delinquent are also regarded as people who are sick. People who constantly flout social conventions are likely to be defined as mentally disturbed. Medicine is, in this sense, an institution of normative coercion (Turner 1995a; Turner and Rojek 2001). We must be attentive to the political implications of medicine, that is, for its impact on social and human rights. Medical sociology recognizes the positive importance of medicine to our lives, but it is also alert to the negative and potentially damaging role of medicine as a social force in the political and moral domain.

Medical sociology came into existence as a branch of sociological theory and research in the early 1950s, with the development of the concept of the sick role, in which sociologists studied the social expectations that define being sick (Cockerham 1986). When a person is sick, there are social expectations that he or she will not work, stay at home, and attempt to get better. Being sick is effectively not being at work. This research treated the social relations between patient and doctor as a "social system" (Parsons 1951). When doctors meet patients, two very different worlds come together, namely, a professional world that is organized hierarchically in terms of a division of labor and a lay world with its own culture and social structure (Maynard 1991; Northouse and Northouse 1987; Rogers 1999). The study of the tensions and conflicts between these two systems has been the central issue of medical sociology for fifty years. It has produced a wealth of information and insight, and it is an extremely rich resource of sociological knowledge about how the social world is organized. However, this microworld of doctor-patient interaction can be understood only within a macro context of medical organization that includes insurance, medical education, professional status, and legal relations. A critical understanding of the doctor-patient relationship requires a more general understanding of both the history of medicine as an institution and its place within society as a whole.

While conventional medical sociology has been specifically

concerned with doctor-patient interactions, we need to sustain a sociological understanding of other equally important questions about social inequality with respect to mortality and morbidity. Why do some social groups live longer and enjoy healthier lives than other social groups? How can we explain the differentials in health and illness between neighborhoods and communities? Why do people in Japan live longer than people in the United States? In order to answer these questions, sociologists need to engage in research in demography and epidemiology or, more generally, in the field of "social medicine." Medical sociology as a special subfield of sociology started in the 1950s with the study of the sick role, but it also has important historical roots in social surveys of poverty and sickness in nineteenth-century cities. In this sense, medical sociology has a broader and larger intellectual history because it has been part of the movement for social medicine and public health.

Social medicine was a reform movement in the nineteenth century that attempted to show how social and economic relations (especially poverty) determined health and illness. Along with the study of public health, it examined how the deprivations of urban industrial society contributed to, or indeed determined, the poor health status of the working class. There has been a long tradition of empirical work to demonstrate that low wages, inadequate housing, hazardous working conditions, poor diet, and deficient sanitation have explained the differences in life expectation between social classes. Social medicine has been critical because it promotes the idea of preventive medicine and social reform as the most adequate response to health issues. It is less concerned with the therapeutic treatment of individuals and more concerned with the transformation of society in order to prevent sickness and disease. Furthermore, social medicine argues that medical treatment of individuals—for example, by vaccination—can be effective only after social reform has already improved sanitation, water supply, food, and housing.

This book is inspired by the legacy of social medicine because I propose that the achievement of social citizenship is a precondition for effective medical intervention to treat the conditions that adversely beset individuals. Social citizenship refers to the rights and entitlements that citizens enjoy either because they have made contributions to society through work, military service, parenting, or other social activities or because governments recognize that they have needs that can be satisfied only collectively. The social rights of citizenship are the legitimate claims that people can make on society for support during periods of hardship and illness. In societies like Britain, Germany, and Sweden, the welfare state has traditionally provided welfare and health benefits to its citizens on a universal basis. In the United States, health and welfare services have not been provided by the state, and individuals have been encouraged to depend on private insurance and philanthropy. My argument is that where health is regarded as a social right, individual health standards improve and health inequality between individuals decreases. Improvements in health take place when there is a general improvement in economic and social conditions. Within such a framework, medical sociology is a critical discipline because it recognizes that the transformation of society is the precondition for the health of individuals. Within a broader international framework, improvements in health are closely related to the promotion and protection of the human rights of individuals and groups (Heggenhougen 2000).

Social medicine has been critical of the health consequences of an unregulated economy and social inequality. In the 1960s and 1970s, critical perspectives on medicine were shaped by radical sociology. The work of Vicente Navarro (1976, 1986) was important in developing the argument that the principal cause of sickness in an industrial capitalist society is the economic exploitation of workers and the impoverishment of their social and cultural lives. Not only are workers exposed to hazards at work, but their life chances are also diminished by their underlying economic exploitation. Navarro's criticisms produced an important research tradition that compared different societies to measure the impact of capitalist relations of production on health—for example, in terms of infant mortality. There is considerable support for Navarro's thesis. For example, the research of Richard G. Wilkinson (1996) has explored the relationships between social inequality, social integration, and health outcomes. Through a series of comparative studies, his research shows that more egalitarian societies have higher levels of social cohesion, lower levels of social disruption, and lower levels of individual stress. As a result, individuals in those societies enjoy better health and live longer, more satisfying lives. There appear to be causal connections between social order, participation, equality, and health.

SOCIAL CAPITAL AND HEALTH

The radical debate about the negative impact of unregulated capitalism on health, inspired by Navarro's research, was an important aspect of sociology in the 1970s, especially in Latin America and Europe (Turner 1995a). Empirical research demonstrated how harsh working conditions in the capitalist economies had serious consequences for the health of workers and their families. With the decline of Communism, however, and the rise of globalization, interests have changed. Gender, age, and lifestyle were seen to be significant determinants of health, and the sociology of social class went into decline. It is possible, however, to defend the core of Navarro's argument, which is that social relations, not the characteristics of individuals, are central to the explanation of health and illness. This thesis presents a challenge to conventional medicine, which concentrates on biological causes, personal therapy, and individualized medicine rather than on social causes, preventive medicine, and collective political responses. In contemporary sociology, as we will discover in later chapters, this type of argument comes under the broader notion of social capital as a more sophisticated measure of social cohesion and integration (Lomas 1998). *Social capital* refers to the "investments" that people make in society, such as their membership in clubs, churches, and associations. The more people have invested in society, the higher their social integration and inclusion in society. The more people are included in society, the less they experience isolation, depression, and illness. In short, the better the social capital of society, the better the health of its individual members. This critical dimension of medical sociology can now be expressed as a theory of social capital, and it provides an alternative to what we might call the neoconservative theory of economics and health (Turner 2003a). My aim in this book is to draw on the ideas of social capital theories and hence to develop a distinctively sociological—rather than a behavioral, psychological, or economic—view of health and illness.

David Coburn (2000) has emphasized the importance of political debate about health and welfare. His approach to health draws on the political sociology of Robert Putnam (1993), especially the notions of social capital and trust. On a global scale, neoconservative economics has reduced the authority of the nation-state, increased social inequality, reduced social cohesion, and diminished social capital. Societies that have low social capital tend to be high in urban decay, interpersonal violence, low confidence in government, and low social trust. Where the social environment is poor and inadequate, there is less protection against infection and disease, and class gradients will increase. This model attempts to connect the decline in social capital with the erosion of the urban environment, loss of self-esteem, and increasing exposure to infection and disease. Individual experiences of health and illness are connected to macro changes in the political environment through concepts of social isolation and social disorganization. This argument can be understood fully only within a global context. The negative effects of unregulated economic markets have been largely borne by poor countries ("the global south"), where debt, disease, and poverty have increased the movement of refugees, economic migrants, and asylum seekers to the rich countries ("the global north") (Sassen 1999). In turn, the growth of global labor markets, migrant networks, tourism, and transportation systems has ensured that infectious diseases are spread more effectively and rapidly. Sociological research on health and illness shows clearly the important connections between social welfare and the health of individuals. The erosion of the social rights of individuals leaves them exposed to the vagaries of rapid economic change, industrial hazard, political instability, and environmental pollution.

BODY AND SOCIETY

While medical institutions are subject to considerable social and political criticism, medicine is clearly an extremely prestigious and powerful institution, partly because the scientific knowledge behind medical practice has enjoyed considerable success in the form of biological inquiry—the human genome project and the cloning of the sheep Dolly are perhaps the most obvious—indeed, spectacular—illustrations. These scientific innovations and developments have placed the human body at the forefront of political and moral controversy (A. W. Frank 1990). The debate about the human body has, in popular discussion, concentrated on topics that raise major moral questions. In terms of media debate, the new reproductive technologies, cloning, and genetic screening are the best illustrations of public concern with the consequences of the "new genetics" (Richards 1993). Improvements in the scientific understanding of genetics have already had major consequences for the conditions under which people reproduce, and genetic surveillance and forensic genetics may transform criminal investigation and the policing of society. It is hardly surprising that the body has become a major concern of modern sociology, giving rise to a new subfield, the sociology of the body (Turner 1984, 1996).

In this study, I have been particularly interested in the social philosophy of Michel Foucault, who has been important in the development of the sociological understanding of the body (Jones and Porter 1994; Petersen and Bunton 1997). Foucault's perspective is useful because he described a division between the study of the individual body and the study of populations (Foucault 1980a). In the first distinction, which he referred to as "an anatomo-politics of the human body," Foucault (1979, 139) examined how various forms of discipline of the body have regulated individuals. In the second distinction, which he referred to as "a bio-politics of the population," Foucault (1979, 139) studied the regulatory controls over populations. Anatomo-politics is concerned with the micropolitics of identity and concentrates on the sexuality, reproduction, and life histories of individuals. The clinical inspection of individuals is part of the anatomo-politics of society. The anatomo-politics of medicine involves the discipline of individuals. The biopolitics of populations uses demography and epidemiology to examine and manage whole populations. The bio-politics of society achieves a surveillance and regulation of populations. Foucault's study of the body was thus organized around the notions of discipline and regulatory controls, or "governmentality." This conceptual framework is parallel to the notions of institutions and normative coercion that I use in this chapter to describe medicine as a social phenomenon.

Medical sociology is particularly concerned with "the government of the body" (Turner 1982), which in modern society involves therapeutic cloning, organ transplants, tissue exchange, organ harvesting, and new reproductive technologies. But the sociology of the body also takes us back to the problems of classical economics and politics, namely, questions about power and scarcity. Perhaps the obvious thing to notice about these corporeal processes and exchanges is that they involve problems of scarcity: the scarcity of viable organs or the scarcity of patients who can afford the operations. In a modern society, human body parts operate, like other commodities, in markets where the laws of supply and demand determine price. These market conditions have not always applied. Take the example of blood donation. Blood may be collected according to a variety of systems, but there are important differences between blood as a gift, blood as a loan, and blood as a commodity. There is a contrast between blood as a gift and blood sold under market conditions (Titmuss 1970). The free market in blood may create an available supply, but it cannot guarantee quality without some regulation. For instance, the gift of blood avoids the problem of addicts' attempting to sell their blood to support their addictions. From a sociological perspective, the problems of scarcity give rise to queues, and in medicine, moral judgments about treatment and supply are unavoidable. For example, does a young alcoholic have a greater claim to a kidney donation than an elderly Methodist teetotaler? Making medical judgments in a setting of scarcity involves moral or value assumptions about the value or worth of patients, and these conditions have an important impact on the uncertainty of medical decision making (R. Fox 1957, 2000). In this study, these forms of social scarcity are described as moral queues because they involve value judgments about the people we regard as worthy of medical treatment.

These issues about scarcity and the politics of the body are particularly acute in the study of aging and dependency, disability and impairment, reproduction and sexuality, and finally, dying and death. In Britain, it has become evident that scarcities within the National Health Service (NHS) have meant that elderly patients are typically at the end of such moral queues and that there is an implicit ranking of patients by age criteria. Because this study is particularly concerned with the issue of the body in society, the processes of aging provide powerful illustrations of my dominant concerns. With the aging of the population, there is an increase in chronic illness and disability, and hence there is demographic pressure on the social distribution of resources to the elderly. The distribution of resources in turn raises important questions about people's entitlements to medical services. The political debate about the relationship between rights, the human body, and disability illustrates many of the questions that are central to medical sociology.

Issues about health and illness are moral and political because health is implicitly employed to describe normality. The problem is that "normality" is variable, contested, and context dependent. Sociologists have emphasized the cultural variability of attitudes toward disability and its role in stigmatization and exclusion. Erving Goffman (1964) distinguished between a stigma of the body (deformities), a stigma of character (alcoholism), and a stigma of social membership (stigmatic groups). Stigma functions to increase social solidarity through a process of social closure. From this perspective, disability is less a matter of physical impairment and more a social process of exclusion. In a society where the body has become a project that defines the moral and social status of the individual, disability has achieved a new level of symbolic importance. Physical impairment and social disability tend to increase with aging. Because aging is an important social aspect of disability, it may be important to recognize the universality of disability

(Zola 1988). There is, as a result, systematic tension between arguments that are sensitive to individual differences and arguments that emphasize social justice and equality. Medical judgments about impairment involve technical or scientific understanding, but they cannot avoid the problem of disability, which in turn presents issues of social rights.

In order to understand the problems associated with an increase in chronic illness and disability, we need to consider the demographic structure of modern societies. Classical economic thought was associated with the demographic theories of Thomas Robert Malthus. After the Second World War, there was a widespread assumption that the world population would follow the demographic revolution that had been common to northern Europe since 1800. The growth of the world population appeared to falsify the basic assumptions of Malthusian political economy. Malthus, in his 1798 *Essay on the Principle of Population, As It Affects the Future Improvement of Society,* argued that given the sexual drive, the need for food, and the declining yield of the soil, the increase in population must overtake the supply of food. Population increase could be controlled by positive means (famine, disease, and war) or preventive means (vice, chastity, and late marriage). In sociological terms, Malthusianism argues that improving the living conditions of the working class cannot be sustained in the long term because it will increase the population, thereby reducing living standards by reducing the food supply. The history of population growth in the United Kingdom does not at first sight support Malthus's theory. The factors that prevented a Malthusian catastrophe were the invention of contraception in the 1820s, the expansion of the food supply through colonialism, and technical improvements in agricultural production. The thesis of a demographic transition asserts that high birth rates and death rates characterize traditional societies—hence their populations tend to be relatively stable. With improvements in nutrition, food supply and distribution, water supply, sanitation, and housing, the death rate falls. These social changes produce an S-shaped population increase. As contraception becomes available and attitudes toward family formation change, the birth rate declines, and the population returns to equilibrium (in the absence of migration and immigration). In Europe, the death rate was declining by the late eighteenth century. By the eve of the Second World War, northern Europe and North America had low fertility rates. The demographic revolution is measured by S-shaped population growth rates.

There has been a corresponding epidemiological transition. In traditional societies, the principal causes of death are infectious diseases (tuberculosis, whooping cough, measles, diphtheria, scarlet fever, and smallpox), especially among infants. The demographic transition produces population aging (because birth rates decline and people live longer); hence, the causes of mortality change to "geriatric diseases" (stroke, heart disease, cancer, and diabetes). In the 1840s in England and Wales, just under three thousand people per million died of tuberculosis; in the late twentieth century, only ten did. While from a public health point of view these changes have primarily social causes (improvements in sanitation, housing, food, and education), the years from 1941 to 1951 were a golden decade of medical advancement in antimicrobial drugs (penicillin, streptomycin, and sulfa drugs) that further reduced the impact of acute infectious sickness. It is important to keep in mind that age-specific causes of death vary considerably from place to place. In the United States, for example, the principal causes of death for men under thirty-five are motor vehicle accidents, suicide, and homicide. In the 1960s, medical sociologists argued that chronic disease was the major issue facing the developed nations and that there was little immediate expectation of dramatic changes in life expectancy. Although chronicity (the prevalence of geriatric diseases) is a major economic and social problem in advanced societies, there has also been a remarkable growth in infectious disease, such as HIV/AIDS and SARS (severe acute respiratory syndrome), since the 1980s as a result of globalization.

In order to understand health and illness sociologically, we need to grasp the relationship between historical changes in the epidemiological causes of morbidity and mortality, the macro-economic environment, and the distribution of scarce resources in society. In order to understand the pattern of health and illness in society, we need to appreciate how the social environment has an impact on the human body. This argument is pursued through an examination of the way global changes in social capital have experiential and corporeal consequences for the individual. The sociology of the body attempts to understand how large-scale changes in the social environment, such as changes in social capital, social order, and citizenship, have consequences for the health and illness of the individual. Improvements in the health of individuals cannot be achieved simply with improvements in medical science without expanding the access of individuals to social resources. The redistribution of resources in society cannot take place without preserving and expanding the social entitlements of citizens.

There are, therefore, complex causal connections between changes in the global economy, changes in social capital, changes in citizenship, and changes in health. Individuals inherit a genetic legacy that predisposes them to risk of specific conditions, but this legacy is always mediated by social circumstances, such as the level of social inequality and social disruption in society. Disease is filtered through the protective network of social capital and citizenship, which mitigate the impact of both genetic legacy and social inequality. Medical sociology therefore has to operate at two levels: analyzing the social structure and describing individual experiences of health and illness. To comprehend these complex relationships between global processes and individual experiences, we need a new medical sociology.

THE NEW MEDICAL SOCIOLOGY

SOCIAL FORMS OF HEALTH AND ILLNESS

Chapter One
HEALTH AND SOCIAL CAPITAL

INTRODUCTION: SOCIAL CITIZENSHIP, RESOURCES, AND HEALTH

WHEN WE GO to a doctor's office with troublesome symptoms, such as a headache, temperature, stiff joints, and runny nose, we are typically given a diagnosis that refers to a natural cause or agent, such as a viral infection; we have influenza. For a range of problems, such diagnostic conclusions are perfectly appropriate, but for problems relating to anxiety, stress, despair, depression, loneliness, or frustration, the causes are more complex, diverse, and uncertain. The outcomes are equally unpredictable. We may feel depressed because we are old and lonely. We may feel unhappy because we believe our bodies are fat and out of control. For such conditions, there is no discrete and specific cause for which medicine has a precise cure. Medical science has not traditionally included social and cultural causes in its diagnostic repertoire, yet there is ample evidence that, for example, that ethnicity, income, education, gender, marital status, and neighborhood play important roles in the distribution of morbidity and mortality in society. In an advanced society, lifestyle plays a significant part in the development and treatment of chronic conditions such as obesity (Hansen 2001).

Sociologists are interested in social involvement (social

capital) and social isolation (estrangement) as key elements in the social causes of health and illness (Turner 2003a). In this connection, the Roseto community public health study is often evoked as an important illustration of how the degree of social integration explains individual health outcomes. In the 1950s and 1960s, it was found that in Roseto, a small Italian American community in Pennsylvania, heart attacks were 50 percent lower than in four surrounding communities. The lifestyles in these communities were similar in terms of smoking, fat intake, diet, and exercise, but Roseto had a tradition of church participation, strong family and social ties, and a high rate of intra-ethnic marriage (Lasker, Egolf, and Wolf 1994). In short, Roseto had a high level of social cohesion or integration. The sociological conclusion is that social membership and social participation act as a buffer against disease. By contrast, social disintegration and social isolation have negative health consequences. Similar community studies by sociologists comparing cohorts for health outcomes have demonstrated that loneliness is bad for our health. James J. Lynch (1977) compared the Roseto study with cohort studies of the town of Framingham, Massachusetts, which also enjoyed good health outcomes and social stability. In a nine-year follow-up, an Alameda County, California, study showed that men and women with few social ties and connections were between two and three times more likely to die than were people with emotionally supportive social networks (S. L. Berkman and Syme 1979). A variety of community-based studies following the Alameda County survey have confirmed the association between social integration and mortality rates (L. F. Berkman 1995). The data from epidemiology, community health studies, and public health research confirm the sociological perspective, which argues that it is the properties of social networks rather than the characteristics of the individuals in them that explain behavior—in this case, the health outcomes of individuals who do or do not have social ties. The social structure appears to act as a shield between the genetic and behavioral characteristics of individuals and their health status.

It is important to note that individuals do not necessarily or consciously choose their social environment. The individuals of the Roseto community and Alameda County did not decide to live in Roseto or Alameda for health reasons and were not aware of the health benefits of social cohesion. In other words, the health outcomes of the individuals were the unintended consequences of the social networks that had been created by marriage and religion. The health consequences were "social facts" and not "individual facts." In this chapter, I want to show how these sociological explanations of health and illness as social facts about the social structure are consistent with the sociological tradition of Émile Durkheim, whose 1897 study of *Suicide* (1951) laid the foundations for theories of social capital in contemporary medical sociology. But we cannot remain entirely content with Durkheim's sociological theory; it requires some extension and modification.

Health is a desirable state of affairs because it is a scarce resource ("a good"). Health, like income, is unequally distributed through the population, but the distribution is not random. Age, ethnicity, gender, income, residence, and status significantly influence the incidence and distribution of health. From a sociological point of view, health is a function of our location within the system of social stratification. This definition is simply one way of saying that health is in part a consequence of social inequality as measured by income, status, educational attainment, gender, and so forth. Our health partly depends on what resources we possess to protect or enhance our well-being. Patterns of health and inequality can be seen in societies where high-income professional groups enjoy longer, healthier lives than low-income low-status groups that have few educational or cultural resources (Macintyre 1997; Wilkinson 1996). Communities or groups that cannot muster social resources to impose social control are exposed to the negative consequences of crime, violence, and social disruption. There are also important comparative differences, whereby many developing African and Asian societies have comparatively high rates of infant mortality that are explained by poverty, poor sanitation, lack of medical facilities, low educational achievement, and social disruption—often resulting from war, ethnic conflict, and civil violence. The declining health of many Central and East European societies, resulting from the social and economic uncertainty of post-Communist economies, provides a clear illustration of the negative effects of social disruption and disorganization on individual health (Hertzman and Siddiqi 2000).

Comparative research in development studies has shown a profound and persistent relationship between poverty and illness, but we need to state this relationship with more precision. The real issue is not poverty but inequality. The best health outcomes are found not necessarily in the richest societies but in the most egalitarian (Wilkinson 1999). Very rich societies are often very unequal societies in which the general level of health is modest. Both the United States and Great Britain are economically rich, but their health statistics reveal often-poor outcomes as measured by infant mortality rates and life expectancy. By contrast, societies with a cultural and political commitment to egalitarianism are societies in which the general quality of social life is positive. Societies that are profoundly unequal also tend to be societies with high levels of urban crime, homicide, civil violence, and low trust. Cross-sectional studies of social capital and violence (homicide and violent crime) in the United States between 1974 and 1993 demonstrated a statistical but nonlinear and dynamic association between inequality and violence (Galea, Karpati, and Kennedy 2002). A "culture of inequality"—characterized by weak social networks, domestic conflict, low trust, alcoholism, and aggression—is manifest in communities with high violence and poor health (Wilkinson 1999, 493). We can treat social citizenship as a set of social and political conditions that enhance an egalitarian distribution of resources and promote social participation. Citizenship and human rights therefore have a direct bearing on social capital and health (Mann et al. 1994).

Differences in health and illness are closely connected to differences in material and cultural resources, and differences in resources reflect differences in power. Because power is ultimately about the capacity of social groups to exercise control over the resources of a society, we cannot neglect the role of power in health and the promotion of health. Resources are not just material and economic; they include cultural resources such as education and status. Social capital (social investments in social networks and connections) is also a fundamental resource. Restoring health to individuals and communities is thus about empowerment. The principal mechanism whereby individuals become empowered is through the institutions of citizenship, which we may define as "that set of practices (juridical, political, economic, and cultural) which define a person as a competent member of society, and which as a consequence shape the flow of resources to persons and social groups" (Turner 1993, 2). Citizenship involves some collective redistribution of resources in favor of vulnerable social groups—the elderly, children, minorities, the unemployed, and so forth—that are particularly exposed to the vagaries of the economic marketplace. The nature and the quality of citizenship vary considerably among societies. In Britain, the development of citizenship in the postwar period was closely associated with the creation of social security and the welfare state. In the United States, citizenship is more closely connected to legal status, political entitlement, and voting rights than to welfare, social entitlements, and the reallocation of resources through government intervention.

The right to health care and treatment is a basic entitlement of social citizenship. In many European societies, citizenship and the welfare state have contributed to social solidarity and hence to social capital by mitigating the social causes of illness, such as poverty, class inequality, and restricted social opportunities. From the sociological perspective on social capital, health is the unintended consequence of the social rights of citizenship and not necessarily an intended outcome of medical interventions. Obviously, preventive health, health education, and social security measures improve individuals' social environment and, consequently, their health characteristics. In a democracy, however, the demand for entitlements also tends to become inflationary. Because governments need to win votes from the electorate, governments in a competitive political environment tend to promise medical and educational benefits that they cannot adequately fund. The competition gives rise to "a legitimation crisis" (Habermas 1976), in which political parties compete for electoral support. As social citizenship and entitlements expand in an inflationary spiral, demands for medical and health services increase. As social expectations rise, scarcity is reintroduced because inflationary demands exceed medical and welfare capacities. Consumers of health services will then turn to alternative forms of supply, such as self-help groups, self-medication, and alternative medicine, because they cannot satisfy their health needs in the formal medical marketplace. Over time, medical services tend to become diverse and pluralistic in a medical market that is, especially in the United States, highly competitive, unregulated, and diverse. This pluralism of services is further magnified by the emergence of e-health, which involves the growth of health Web sites from which customers can derive information, medication, and services that do not depend directly on professional medical sources. In order to understand health and illness in modern societies, we need to study the complex interactions of new technologies, social citizenship, social structure, and the politics of resource allocation. The contemporary debate about social capital provides a convenient location for understanding the complex relationships between these different dimensions of the social structure.

DEFINITIONS OF SOCIAL CAPITAL

The contemporary theory of social capital has a number of different intellectual origins, and hence its definition is often unstable. Generic definitions of social capital have been provided by Nan Lin (2001, 29) as "resources embedded in a social structure that are accessed and/or mobilized in purposive actions" and by Alejandro Portes (1998) as the ability to derive benefits from membership of networks and related social structures. Lin proposed that social actors rationally manipulate and exploit their social connections and networks to maximize the return on their social investments. The concept of social capital developed out of economics as a method of explaining economic investments in education, training, and welfare in order to produce human capital. The theory became closely associated with the sociological contribution of James Coleman to the analysis of the social functions of education. In his article "Social Capital in the Creation of Human Capital," Coleman (1988) showed how social capital facilitates social action through trust and trustworthiness. In his *Foundations of Social Theory,* Coleman (1994) treated human capital (such as investment in education) and social capital (the interpersonal relations that facilitate collective action) as complementary. In his analysis of social capital, Coleman used a medical example to explore the relations between obligations and expectations in social life. He observed that in the traditional relationship between patient and family doctor, the physician, in addition to getting paid for his or her services, received the gratification, esteem, and deference of the family, and those intangible dimensions of the social relationship contributed to the physician's high social status. Those obligations that the family invested in the relationship with the physician were social capital. They "inhibited patients dissatisfied with the outcome of their medical treatment from taking action against their physician" (308). With the economic transformation of medicine, the traditional family doctor has largely disappeared, the status of the physician has declined relative to the patients, and the patients are more likely to see a specialist than a general practitioner. Finally, the increased use of liability insurance transfers liability from physicians to insurers. The result is a decline in the social capital that protected doctors from becoming targets of patients dissatisfied with their health outcomes.

Recently, the theory of social capital has been closely associated with political sociology through Robert Putnam's study of the conditions of democracy. His theory is distinctive because it attempts to demonstrate the relationship between trust and social connectedness. In *Making Democracy Work*, Putnam (1993) showed that civil society cannot function without social trust, and trust arises from two sources, namely the norms of reciprocity and networks of civic engagement. We tend to trust people when we think they are following the implicit and explicit rules of behavior that are prevalent in the community. These rules are the "norms of reciprocity" that make social life run smoothly. When people spontaneously adhere to local rules and customs, we do not need to rely overtly on police intervention to regulate our neighbors. They are committed to making the community work, and hence they are involved in these networks of social engagement. Society "works" because high levels of trust mean that we will not need to depend explicitly on law enforcement agencies to get things done.

In *Bowling Alone*, Putnam (2000) demonstrated that in America the generation that grew up with television after the Second World War had relatively few associational ties and that social capital was declining. With the erosion of social capital, there was also a troublesome decline in trust. Social life became difficult because as trust declined, individuals felt they could not rely on people to get things done. Social activities require more effort, and hence we can argue that social capital or trust makes social engagements more efficient. When I cannot trust my surgeon to look after me during an operation, I am forced to invest a lot of effort in taking out insurance policies, getting a second opinion, seeking alternative advice from complementary medicine, or checking on the surgeon's record with previous patients. In an extreme situation, I may be forced to ask the hospital for his or her surgical records: how many patients died on the operating table under unusual circumstances? Trust is the social oil that makes society flow smoothly.

Putnam's approach to social capital has consequently been extended in social science to make comparisons with the idea of human capital as an essential aspect of economic development (Dasgupta 1993; Dasgupta and Serageldin 2000). His work has been important in political debates about the decline of social capital in American public life, where his theories have been associated with the legacy of Alexis de Tocqueville, who in 1835, in *Democracy in America* (1968), argued that voluntary associations are the bedrock of American democratic culture. Putnam's research is particularly important for medical sociology because he demonstrated that the decline in social capital has a negative impact on health.

The idea that social capital involves investments in voluntary associations has been taken from the work of Tocqueville, who in the early nineteenth century observed that the prominence of voluntary associations was the most astonishing feature of American social life. Whereas people in Europe were dependent on the state for many essential services, local communities in postcolonial America would create voluntary groups to develop civic buildings, construct roads, build schools, or found hospitals. Writing in 1831, Tocqueville (1959, 212) argued that the "power of the association had reached its highest degree in America," where it served many purposes, but "[t]he last word in the way of any association seems to me to be the temperance societies, that is to say an association of men who mutually agree to abstain from vice, and find in collective power an aid in resisting what is most intimate and personal to each man, his own inclinations."

Tocqueville's ideas on democracy have been invigorated by Putnam's research into civic traditions in America and Italy, in which he concluded that social capital is a feature of social organization that includes trust, norms, and networks that "can improve the efficiency of a society by facilitating co-ordinated actions" (1993, 167). Social trust is essential for building up civil society through norms of reciprocity and engagement, and it is the main antidote to the negative effects of individual greed and egoism that are characteristic of markets in modern societies. Social capital represents the investments of people in communal activity.

These different approaches to social participation and trust can be summarized by defining social capital as the social investments of individuals in society in terms of their membership in formal and informal groups, networks, and institutions. Social capital therefore provides us with an objective measure of the degree of social integration or social solidarity in any society. The density of the social membership of community groups, churches, parent associations, voluntary associations, and neighborhood groups is a measure of the extent of reciprocity and an index of the vitality of trust. Social isolation and alienation from social connections are obviously negative indices of social cohesion and social capital. The social capital debate about the macrofoundations of health locates the underlying problem of health and illness in the social distribution of resources through effective forms of citizenship. It is important to recognize that the social capital debate has emerged as a critical tool to analyze the negative effects of growing social inequality on global health in a period of neoconservative economic reform.

ÉMILE DURKHEIM AND THE STUDY OF SUICIDE

In the social science literature, social capital theory often assumes two characteristic features that locate it within a primarily economic vision of social action: rational choice and individualism. In Nan Lin's theory of social capital, individuals consciously and rationally manipulate their investments in social networks to maximize their benefits. These are not typically sociological assumptions. For example, in the Roseto case study, individuals do not necessarily regard marriage or church membership as a rational strategy to maximize their health status. Sociological explanations often involve explanations of the effects of social structure on outcomes about which the social actors themselves may be ignorant or poorly informed. Sociology does not deny human agency or consciousness; indeed, it insists that action as opposed to behavior requires agency and consciousness. However, sociology pays particular attention to the unintended consequences of social action. The lower incidence of heart disease in Roseto is an interesting illustration of the unintended consequences of communal solidarity arising from high levels of intermarriage, church membership, and social participation.

This approach to social capital was first developed at the turn of the century by the French sociologist Émile Durkheim in two major publications, one on suicide and one on civil society. Durkheim never used the phrase *social capital,* but his notions of social solidarity and social facts are useful in developing a sociological understanding of health and illness from the perspective of social connectedness and civil society (L. F. Berkman et al. 2000). Durkheim argued against the legacy of the late-nineteenth-century British evolutionary sociologist Herbert Spencer, according to which the wave of suicide in nineteenth-century France was a consequence of egoistic individualism, the erosion of moral sanctions on individuals, unpredictable business cycles, and the decline of civil groups and institutions. In *Suicide,* Durkheim (1951) showed that suicide rates increased when social integration and social regulation declined. He identified four types of suicide (egoistic, anomic, altruistic, and fatalistic) and showed how they relate to social integration and social regulation. Young men in an urban setting, without religious and familial connections, experienced a greater exposure to suicidal pressures than Catholic parents in stable rural communities. Two types of suicide, egoistic and anomic, have dominated the secondary literature on suicide in sociology because they most clearly illustrate Durkheim's criticisms of modern society. Anomic suicide is common where the inflated expectations of modern life lead, through economic crises, to disappointment and despair. For Durkheim, the decline of religious and moral constraints on individuals has left them fully exposed to the suicidal currents of modern society.

Durkheim is often regarded as a conservative social theorist because in many of his explanations the decline of religion causes social disruption and disorganization. In fact, Durkheim did not believe that a restoration of religious authority was likely in modern society, and he argued that social integration would require the intervention of the state as a moral institution and the restoration of civil society through associations. In *Professional Ethics and Civic Morals,* Durkheim (1992) argued that the intermediary ties between individuals and the state were being eroded, and hence the individual was increasingly isolated and detached from the intermediary social groups and associations of civil society. Durkheim's theory of intermediary groups is analytically connected to Tocqueville's theory of voluntary associations, and we must assume that Durkheim had studied Tocqueville's political sociology of associations.

Social capital theory indicates that social involvement protects individuals from episodes of sickness and from psychological depression. Contemporary research examining the relationship between social capital and depression can be regarded as a contemporary application of Durkheim's theory of suicide, in which individuals are protected from suicidal forces by the density of their social relationships.

Durkheim's contribution to social capital theory has received scant recognition. Durkheim (1951, 299) argued that there exists "for each people a collective force of a definite amount of energy, impelling men to self-destruction." We can imagine social capital acting as a social shield against stress, accident, and disease. Durkheim's approach was characteristic of early sociological research on depression. For example, George Brown's work was particularly important in providing an explanation of the differential experience of depression in men and women. George W. Brown and Tirril Harris (1978) demonstrated that women, who represent two-thirds of all cases of clinical depression in Britain, suffered from a number of psychological and social adversities and deprivations that could produce depression. The causal factors of depression (or vulnerability factors) were the loss of a mother before eleven years of age, lack of employment, and three or more children under the age of fourteen at home. The most important protection against such depressive forces was the presence of an intimate friendship or social relationship. This research can be interpreted to say that social investments (employment and friendships) are the best protection against depression. Contemporary research from various societies shows that social support and good social networks, especially for women, are associated with lower scores on psychological symptoms of depression (Kuh et al. 2002).

Durkheim's studies of suicide and civil society provide the fertile theoretical ground in classical sociology that indicates an important relationship between social involvement (social capital), intermediary institutions and associations, and individual well-being (health). Durkheim's analysis of suicide and his causal model have, however, been heavily criticized. For example, his analysis of suicide rates has been regarded as too mechanistic in the sense that individual suicide is a consequence of suicidal forces driving to self-destruction an individual who has become disconnected from society. Despite sustained criticism,

Durkheimian sociology is enjoying a remarkable revival (Pickering 2002), which is evident in the debate about declining health and the politics of neoconservatism. In addition, comparative social research has consistently supported Durkheim's causal analysis of youth suicide. Richard Eckersley and Keith Dear (2002), noting the worldwide increase in suicide rates among young men over the last fifty years, commented that the rise in suicide reflects the failure of developed societies to provide appropriate sources of identity and attachment while encouraging inappropriate expectations about individual freedom and autonomy. These findings are consistent with Durkheim's analysis of individualism, isolation, and disappointment. Durkheim was a major critic of the English tradition of utilitarian individualism, arguing that there was no convincing evidence that economic individualism produced an increase in happiness. It is ironic that there should be a Durkheimian revival directed against the global consequences of neoconservatism for health and well-being.

In the new-millennium issue of *Social Science & Medicine*, the "neo-Durkheimian approach" to health and inequality was recognized as an important development because "social capital concepts such as group membership, social trust or degree of social cohesion are shown to be associated with health status at the macro level, and mediate the relationship between income inequality and health" (Blaxter 2000, 1140). The sudden collapse of the Soviet Union and its satellites in Eastern Europe has produced a social laboratory within which social scientists have measured the impact of declining social capital, in terms of increases in crime and political conflict, on higher mortality rates and lower self-assessed health (Kawachi, Kennedy, and

Wilkinson 1999). This post-Communist experiment provides a unique opportunity to test Durkheim's theory of social disruption and its consequences as measured by crime, violence, alcoholism, prostitution, and poor health (Cockerham 2000). The essence of the Durkheimian view of society is that the isolated individual, in times of rapid social change and social disruption, is subject to social forces that can destroy his or her mental and physical well-being. Individual isolation and social dislocation are, not surprisingly, important causes of physical and mental distress. Gerry Veenstra (2000), in an important Canadian study, found that as measures of social engagement, frequency of socialization with workmates and attendance at religious services had the strongest positive relationship with health from a battery of indicators. The negative relationship between isolation and poor health is well-known, and socially isolated individuals tend to reside in neighborhoods with low social capital (L. F. Berkman and Glass 2000). These studies generally confirm the Durkheimian theory that low social integration and poor social regulation expose individuals to "social currents" that result in mental instability and physical illness.

The Durkheimian revival has many dimensions and has been employed to explain both mental and physical health and illness. Durkheim's idea that social integration protects individuals from episodes of psychological depression was applied to community studies of mental health. Social psychologists studied how community and social ties provided social integration that guarded against the impact of negative life events (Dohrenwend and Dohrenwend 1981). Further research explored how social support might more directly act as a buffer against serious life events, such as divorce and bereavement

(S. L. Berkman and Syme 1979). While psychologists have been aware of the impact of stress on individual health, it is difficult to find objective measures of stress to explain variance in health outcomes. Life events provide an alternative measure of episodes that attack an individual's composure and self-esteem. Stress and strain in social relations are obviously related to the life cycle, and the decline of "relational stress" with aging may compensate for the eventual decline in social participation that is an inevitable feature of the aging process (Due et al. 1999). We have already noted that psychological research on young, isolated women suffering from depression provides an illustration of the value of Durkheimian sociology. In addition, G. W. Brown and Harris (1978) demonstrated that social structures, primarily friendship networks, protect vulnerable individuals, typically young mothers, from the depressive effects of negative life events. Durkheim's idea of suicidal currents blindly driving individuals to suicide has been refined to demonstrate that individuals do not necessarily succumb to "depressive forces" if they are socially integrated into primary social relationships, such as the family or a neighborhood group. Social integration as measured by church involvement has also been shown to be negatively associated with depressive symptoms (Latkin and Curry 2003). This argument can be summarized to claim that high social capital means that individuals are protected from episodes of mental illness. Does the same argument apply to physical health, and what are the precise connections between social structures and individual behavior?

An extensive literature in the social sciences demonstrates that membership in voluntary organizations contributes to a decrease in psychological stress and protects against the principal forms of stress (Rietschlin 1998). Voluntary association membership is important in increasing satisfaction and reducing depression and is associated with improvements in physical well-being and lower mortality. The relationship between well-being (both physical and mental) and membership in voluntary associations is likely to be reciprocal and circular because healthy, confident, and satisfied individuals are more likely to join voluntary associations than depressed and alienated individuals. A recent study by Peggy Thoits and Lyndi Hewitt (2001) on "Volunteer Work and Well-Being" confirmed the reciprocal relationship between satisfaction and voluntary association membership, but their focus on work rather than simply membership demonstrated an independent contribution. They discovered that "volunteer service is beneficial to personal well-being independent of other forms of religious and secular community participation" (126). Voluntary work and membership enhance various aspects of well-being, including happiness, physical health, and decreased depression. Active involvement in volunteering appears to have a beneficial effect on the mental health of people over sixty-five years of age by reducing levels of depression. This positive effect among the elderly suggests that voluntary work has a special salience when other forms of social involvement have been reduced (Musick and Wilson 2003).

Social capital theory has been a method of recasting existing theories relating income inequality to individual morbidity and mortality. A long tradition of social science research has employed income inequality as a measure of social class to demonstrate that infant mortality rates, for example, are highly correlated with parental income (Wilkinson 1992). More recent versions of the theory have suggested that income inequality is causally connected to population health via societal variables, namely, social cohesion and trust, and that cohesion and trust are measures of social capital. In the United States, research has taken measurements of trust in individual states to show that trust has a direct effect on the relationship between income inequality and life expectancy (Kawachi et al. 1999). The underlying thesis is that high levels of income inequality in a society produce low trust, and low trust creates a poor social environment, which in turn has an impact on individual health. While low income among low-status men is clearly associated with poor health, the health of low-income men is still improved by the presence of social supports (Antonucci, Ajrouch, and Janevic 2003).

The causal connections that tie social capital to health outcomes have remained controversial. Social capital can be important in the provision of health services and the distribution of medical information to the general public. Communities with high levels of social cohesion are more effective in organizing to sustain or increase access to medical services and amenities than communities with low levels of social cohesion. In their study of internal differences within the United States, epidemiologists found that states with high levels of social cohesion had more egalitarian patterns of political participation, which also ensured better health services for their members (L. F. Berkman and Kawachi 2000). Research on income inequality by households demonstrates significant inequality between states, with Louisiana the most unequal and New Hampshire the most egalitarian (Kaplan et al. 1996). Income inequality was associated not only with higher mortality rates but also with higher rates of premature death, heart disease, and cancer (Kawachi and Kennedy 2002, 103). Sociologists have also found that social capital influences health behaviors by promoting the diffusion of health information and thereby increases the likelihood that healthy lifestyles are adopted. Lisa F. Berkman and her colleagues (2000) have suggested that we examine the links between supportive social networks and beneficial health outcomes through a division between "upstream factors" and "downstream factors." The argument is that upstream factors are the macro social-structural conditions that shape social networks at the meso level. The macro factors embrace both cultural and material conditions, from supportive values to civil wars. The meso level is composed of the quantity of supportive networks and the quality of interpersonal relationships. These macro and meso conditions provide the downstream opportunities, at the micro level, for effective psychosocial mechanisms for psychological satisfaction from social supports, social influence, engagements, and interpersonal connections that have an impact on a variety of pathways to individual health outcomes. These pathways at the micro level include many lifestyle factors, such as smoking, diet, exercise, and help-seeking behavior, and it is at this level that lifestyle connects with behavioral and physiological consequences in terms of immune system functions, cardiovascular reactivity, and cardiopulmonary fitness. Research on survival rates of people who have suffered heart attacks also demonstrates that social supports are crucial. Among patients admitted to the hospital with heart attacks, 38 percent who reported having no social or emotional support died in the hospital, compared with almost 12 percent who had two or more supports (L. F. Berkman, Leo-Summers, and Horwitz 1992). In another study, patients who had poor social support and were isolated were more than twice as likely to die over a three-year period than patients with strong social networks (Case, Moss, and Case 1992). Psychosomatic studies of human and nonhuman populations (such as higher primates) indicate that poor social relationships characterized by aggression and isolation result in negative cellular immune responses (L. F. Berkman 1995). There is evidence, therefore, that a causal chain linking low social capital to physiological consequences can explain why social cohesion is associated with good health and social isolation with poor health.

There is also evidence that individuals with robust social networks engage in less health-damaging behavior (tobacco and alcohol consumption) than individuals who are socially disconnected (Trieber et al. 1991). Berkman's research on social isolation has produced the important hypothesis that isolation and disconnectedness have an impact on the organism in terms of a process of accelerated aging. In particular, childhood experiences of social deprivation produce accelerated aging when one looks at the individual in terms of the life-course. This research indicates that static models of health behavior are inadequate and that both generational and life-course models offer a more sophisticated framework for sociological research.

Although critics have challenged social capital theory for its methodology, quality of data, and causal argumentation (Fiscella and Franks 1997; Gravelle 1998), research demonstrating the connections between income inequality, social investments, and health is persistent and persuasive. The causal relationship between income inequality at the individual level and aggregate income inequality on health outcomes remains controversial, but recent research has shown that societies with higher aggregate income inequality will always have worse health at the macro level than societies with lower aggregate income inequality because an increase in aggregate social inequality will always have a disproportionately negative effect on the very poor (Robert and House 2000, 127). There is a curvilinear relationship between income and health because as income increases, health improves, but for the rich, increases in income have relatively little impact on health. Increases in aggregate income inequality will reduce healthy outcomes.

DEVELOPMENTS IN SOCIAL CAPITAL THEORY

There is clearly a need to refine the social capital thesis on different dimensions. The debate has been refined theoretically by Penelope Hawe and Alan Shiell (2000), who distinguish between the relational, material, and political aspects of social capital. The relational aspect might be regarded as the Durkheimian, or sociological, dimension and is clearly illustrated by the Roseto case study and similar instances of social science research. Although existing research on social capital and health is interesting and suggestive, we need more evidence from a life-course perspective that will examine how individuals acquire or lose social networks over time. Increasing loneliness is an obvious consequence of aging (Elias 1982), and thus participation in religious services and clubs has a beneficial effect on the health of the elderly (Veenstra 2000).

The political dimension of health and inequality—namely, the issue of power—has been another aspect of the social capital debate. At both the psychological and the social level, the

sense of powerlessness and alienation has been closely impli-
cated in poor mental and physical health. It is in the field of
capacity building and community development, however, that
the notion of social capital as power has had important consequences for social policy. Capacity building for communities
means improving the capacity of residents and their organizations to achieve collective goals and to work together to sustain
programs for urban improvement. These revitalization programs aim to secure a more diverse base for leadership, greater
involvement of residents in local associations, and a widely
shared vision of neighborhood improvement. In effect, community capacity building entails building social capital. There are
critics who see the idea of capacity building as "comprehensive
community initiatives," which can be a romantic or idealistic
vision of community (Kubisch and Stone 2001). For example,
Hawe and Shiell (2000, 879) draw an important distinction
between what they regard as the "romantic essentially middle
class view of social capital" of Robert Putnam and Pierre Bourdieu's idea of social capital as a field of social struggles over influential "connections" (Bourdieu 1993, 32). In talking about
"community" as a source for protecting individuals from risks,
we must recognize that communities are receptacles of power
and that they are stratified by social and cultural capital.
Health interventions for the improvement of capacity building
in communities cannot afford to neglect this dimension of
community power. Social capital is an important bridge between individuals and contributes to the social solidarity of the
community, but it can also act as a barrier between communities. It is for this among other reasons that health and citizenship become entwined politically and sociologically.

Effective and empowered citizens support and are supported by communities that have capacities, and the capacity for action is essentially what Coleman (1994) meant by social capital when he argued that a social group whose members place considerable trust in one another will be able to accomplish collective goals much more effectively than groups with low trust. A society with effective social citizenship will enjoy higher levels of trust because its citizens will be actively involved in social activities and projects. Reserves of social capital will also require effective social policies to improve housing and social services and to control drugs if individuals are to enjoy improvements in health (Latkin and Curry 2003, 41). The new public health perspective (Petersen and Lupton 1996) recognizes the centrality of citizenship to health promotion, but it is also important to acknowledge that there are differences in the historical relationship between citizens and the state. Within a welfare tradition dominated by the state and large corporations, as in Germany, Japan, Russia, and Austria, the citizen can be passive and acquiescent, in which case it is the state that constructs the healthy citizen, but within a liberal communitarian perspective the active citizen contributes to the collective building of public health.

Two rather different versions of social capital theory link income inequality to health. The first attempts to link the psychological responses of individuals in terms of trust and social cohesion to societies in which there is greater social equality (Kawachi and Kennedy 1997). The second argues that income inequality is associated with public investment in aspects of the social infrastructure, such as housing, sanitation, and education (Davey Smith 1996). These material conditions have

direct consequences for individual health independent of socioeconomic position, but their effects are more pronounced
among low-income groups. It is social capital as a material investment in society that explains changes in both crime and
health rates as measures of what Durkheim called "anomie," or
normlessness.

THE NEOCONSERVATIVE ECONOMIC REVOLUTION

The neoconservative economic revolution of the 1970s has had
the consequence of increasing health inequality between and
within societies. Recent sociological research has returned to
the issue of income inequality as an explanation of sickness but
has set income inequalities within the broader context of social
integration and cohesion. This development therefore combines the radical legacy of Karl Marx and political economy
with the sociological legacy of Durkheim. There appears to be
an important connection between the level of aggregate inequality in society, social divisions, the decline of social involvement, low trust, low self-esteem, and increasing morbidity and
declining mortality. High crime rates, social disorganization,
domestic violence, and civil disturbance also indicate low social
capital. Social capital is a method of measuring social integration as social investments. Crudely speaking, the more people
are involved in society, the better they are protected from poor
mental and physical health. In this radical epidemiology, sickness is a function of high inequality and low social cohesion.
The biological and psychological connections between individual health outcomes, social participation, and economic
inequality remain somewhat obscure, but one can reasonably
assume that a sense of self-worth is a consequence of a support-

ive social environment, which in turn has beneficial consequences for the human immune system. Poor social relationships leave their mark on the human body by means of the intermediary of low self-esteem and lack of social support.

The development of "the new public health" (Petersen and Lupton 1996) has coincided with a revival of social epidemiology in terms of a search for research paradigms that can capture the impact of social networks, rather than individual characteristics, on health. These developments involve a return to the origins of the public health movement of the 1840s, which sought to improve the health of individuals by improving the health of society through educational reform, the creation of democratic institutions, and the improvement of the material and social infrastructure. The crisis in health and the increase in crime in Russia and other post-Communist states serve as important evidence of how health is related to individual income inequality and aggregate social disorder (Siegrist 2000). The decline in life expectancy in Russia is a consequence of life chances rather than life choices, a consequence, that is, of aggregate effects of inequality and instability on levels of stress (Cockerham 2000). Post-Communism provides a large but tragic illustration of social anomie and its consequences for individual health.

The debate about social capital within medical sociology has been in part about whether neoconservatism has brought about a new set of macroeconomic conditions or whether the argument merely supports existing findings on the effects of social inequality on health. David Coburn has argued that the neoconservative policies of the 1980s that were designed to increase profitability through global competition and deregulation have increased social inequality and decreased health, especially in developing societies (2000). The conservative revolt against economic regulation in the 1970s became dominant in the 1980s. The neoconservative revolution attempted to show that welfare impedes economic growth, that government services are inefficient and bureaucratic, that states that funded welfare through deficit financing would ultimately fail, and that privatization policies would improve efficiency and profitability. These policies were also based on the assumption that welfare promotes dependency and laziness and that patients should pay user fees. The neoconservative revolution was therefore a sustained attack on the social Keynesianism that had been the basis of social reconstruction in the 1940s and 1950s. Coburn has attempted to demonstrate that these policies have reduced social capital and eroded many health gains. His thesis has been amplified by Alvin Tarlov (2000), who argued that neoconservatism also diminishes state authority and welfare priorities, which reduce social cohesion and increase the population's health gradient. One paradox of neoconservatism was to increase the dependence of the state on voluntary associations, which were expected to form alliances with governments in order to provide a welfare strategy that encouraged participation and independence. The third sector (voluntary associations, charities, and philanthropic groups) has expanded to meet the challenge through various mechanisms, such as competitive bidding for government funding or community enterprise strategies. These voluntary associations have come to be driven by the logic of resource management, and the boundary between for-profit and not-for-profit organizations has become blurred. In short, community enterprise and voluntary associations have become part of a more general enterprise culture (K. Brown, Kenny, and Turner 2000).

There are two major criticisms of Coburn. The first is historical. For example, in Britain, health inequalities widened substantially during the 1950s and 1960s, when the NHS under social Keynesian policies was already established; and thus it cannot be said that increasing social inequality can be confined to periods when neoconservatism is dominant (Wilkinson 2000). Second, Coburn has not identified the causal links between the absence of friendship, low self-esteem, low social status, and poor health. For Richard G. Wilkinson, friendship and social dominance are merely two sides of the same coin. Income inequality is simply one measure of power—that is, of dominance and hierarchy in human societies. The more unequal societies become, the more hierarchical relations between individuals become dominant. The result is an increase not only in homicide, suicide, and aggression but also in anxiety and chronic stress, resulting in sickness and depression. These criticisms suggest that the Coburn thesis on neoconservatism and health merely revisits the existing arguments about the negative effects of social inequality. Other critics of Coburn argue that the globalization process, of which neoconservatism is a part, has had paradoxical benefits, such as the spread of the Internet, which has made top-down, hierarchical control of information impossible. In this argument, the Internet spreads democracy by permitting marginal groups a voice in global politics (Hertzman 2000).

There are various ways in which the Coburn thesis could be defended. In my argument about the new medical sociology, two aspects of Coburn's thesis remain crucial. The first is that social cohesion, or interconnectedness, is a fundamental aspect of health in promoting social trust and well-being (J. W. Lynch 2000). It is clear, however, that we do not fully understand the precise causal mechanisms that connect health and well-being in individuals with social capital via a variety of psychological mechanisms, such as self-esteem, confidence, and happiness. The second is that Coburn's argument points to the fact that a comparative perspective that adopts a society-by-society approach to understanding these global transformations will not constitute a satisfactory and comprehensive sociological understanding of globalization.

These negative features of global neoconservatism have served as the background to the development of social capital theory. Neoconservatism diminishes the authority of the state and makes more difficult the achievement of welfare priorities. At the same time, it increases social inequality and reduces the level of social cohesion (or social capital) in society. These structural changes lower the level of social trust in a society and diminish self-respect in those sectors of the community that are exposed to growing social inequality. Coburn's approach is important because it allows us to make a direct connection between the global growth of neoconservatism, the decline in social cohesion, and the erosion of the health of individuals.

CONCLUSION: SOCIOLOGY AND SOCIAL PATHOLOGY

Durkheim's social theory belongs to a tradition of French political and social analysis that was concerned with the social causes of social pathology in modern societies (Gane 2003). The French Revolution decisively transformed traditional French society and unleashed social forces—secularization, rational administration, democratization, military reform, and educational change—that promoted the formation of modern society. In many respects, sociology as a secular and positive science of society was itself a product of the French Revolution. Upheavals in French society gave rise to the idea that societies are like social organisms that exhibit social pathologies just as natural organisms have diseases. Social philosophers developed various comparisons between medical science and the study of disease on the one hand and social science and the study of social pathology on the other.

Before the development of the term *sociology* in the 1820s, *social physics* was the name given to the study of the laws of the social organism. The early development of sociology was undertaken in the nineteenth century by Auguste Comte, who was significantly influenced by key figures in the development of medical science after the French Revolution, particularly developments in physiology such as those made by Pierre Cabanis, Franz Joseph Gall, and François Broussais (Wernick 2001). Comte recognized that the expansion of medical science had produced a new understanding of the causal determinants of individual human behavior, but human beings were seen as members of a "social species," and it was important to understand the social institutions, language, knowledge, religion, and culture that determined social life. The task of sociology was to understand the structure and processes of the "social organism" and to comprehend the historical stages through which society has evolved. Sociology replaced social physics as the study of the autonomous world of the social order that cannot be reduced to the characteristics of its individual members.

It is obvious that Durkheim's analysis of the methods to be

used in the study of social facts, in *The Rules of Sociological Method* (1964), is a contribution to an intellectual tradition that starts with Comte. First, following Comte, Durkheim defined social facts as "ways of acting, thinking, and feeling, external to the individual, and endowed with a power of coercion, by reason which they control him" (3). In the language of contemporary sociology, we might designate these social facts as social institutions, such as law, religion, and morality. Durkheim also identified a classification of "social currents," such as "great movements of enthusiasm, indignation, and pity in a crowd" (4). It is the task of sociology to explain these social facts not by reference to the characteristics of individuals but by reference to the social structure. Second, Durkheim took up the problem of understanding social pathology. The chapter on the normal and the pathological in *The Rules* is an extensive reflection on the problems of defining health in living organisms and the normal in social systems. Durkheim identified a paradox in pathological processes in both cases: while aging might be regarded as a pathological process, it is a normal aspect of the life process. Similarly, crime is a normal aspect of social life that can enhance respect for and commitment to the law. Although Durkheim recognized that defining normality in social life is problematic, he eventually treated the average as a criterion of the normal: "A social fact is normal, in relation to a given social type at a given phase of its development, when it is present in the average society of that species at the corresponding phase of its development" (64). In *Suicide,* Durkheim argued that suicide was not as such abnormal, but the rapid growth in the suicide rate in Europe in the nineteenth century was indicative of a morbid social condition. The suicide rate "cannot be normal. . . . They result not from a regular evolution but from a morbid disturbance which, while able to uproot the institutions of the past, has put nothing in their place" (1951, 369).

In contemporary sociology, the language of "social pathology" and "morbid disturbance" has largely disappeared, and there is generally a reluctance to make detailed comparisons between biological organisms and social systems. Although the language has changed, there may be important continuities in the sociological objectives of Comte and Durkheim. In this chapter, we have seen how modern sociologists have used Durkheim's approach to argue that social isolation and social disruption are negatively associated with health. Furthermore, the social disorganization that has been associated with the fall of Communism, the globalization of the economy, the impact of civil wars and ethnic conflicts, and the social reforms of neoconservative economic policies has produced a decline in life expectancy and increases in morbidity in many societies. Durkheim argued that the new economic order of nineteenth-century capitalism in France produced the social pathology of an anomic society resulting in abnormal suicide rates. Contemporary social capital theory argues that rapid social and economic change in the late twentieth century produced social isolation and social disorganization ("social pathology"), resulting globally in poor health.

Chapter Two
THE SOCIAL CONSTRUCTION OF KNOWLEDGE

INTRODUCTION: DURKHEIM AND CLASSIFICATION

CONTEMPORARY SOCIOLOGISTS have been critical of Durkheim's conception of social facts. In terms of the suicide rate, Jack D. Douglas (1967) argued that the official statistics on suicide are not reliable because they obscure the complexity of the social processes by which certain deaths are recorded as suicides. In order to understand the social meanings of suicide, sociologists should examine the implicit assumptions that underpin official decisions such as coroners' judgments about suicide notes. Contemporary sociologists are likely to question official data as unreliable, especially for comparative purposes, and take the view that social facts are socially constructed. In this chapter, I shall examine the contributions of social constructionism to medical sociology. Before exploring social constructionism, however, we need to examine Durkheim's approach to social classification.

Durkheim interpreted social facts as aspects of the collective representation of a society. For example, religious beliefs and symbols are representations of the society as a whole. For our purposes, we need to interpret Durkheim's social facts in the context of his sociology of knowledge because Durkheim was above all interested in the problem of social classification. He did not, therefore, treat social facts naively. The main thrust of

Durkheim's theory of classification is that classification is collective and derives its authority from collective processes. Our basic concepts about space and time are social products—they are social representations. Durkheim's sociology of knowledge as a whole was a critical response to the legacy of Immanuel Kant's eighteenth-century epistemology. For Durkheim and his school, classificatory principles are not individualistic, a priori, and rational. In *Primitive Classification* (1963), Durkheim and Marcel Mauss showed that the authority and effectiveness of classification come from the facts that classificatory systems are collective, that they remain vivid as a result of social rituals, that they remain forceful because they draw on collective emotions, and finally that their reality is underpinned by their representation of social structures. Classification works because it is a collective representation, but it requires collective rituals to make it vivid and compelling. The conclusion was that the logical force of a classificatory system is rooted in a collective experience of the sacred. Durkheim thought that in modern society, classification principles, such as the fundamental contrast between the sacred and the profane, had lost their authoritative force because the decline of religion and the rise of individualism had changed the nature of collective life. Hence the classificatory systems of modern societies are weak and unstable. The erosion of classificatory authority means that there is increasing dispute about the meaning of social facts, and hence emerge the social conditions in which people will argue that social facts are socially constructed. The "facticity" of social facts is no longer taken for granted; the classificatory paradigms of society, including medical classifications, become sites of political struggle and contest.

MEDICAL KNOWLEDGE

In modern sociological theory, power and knowledge are closely connected. We can interpret power as the capacity to define social reality in terms of one's own interests. Sociological debates about medical power and knowledge eventually come to focus on two questions: what is a disease, and who has the power to define diseases? In attempting to answer these questions, we are faced with interesting choices: are diseases discovered, are they invented, or are they socially constructed? Let us take an example. We could argue that anorexia nervosa, a psychological condition in which people have a systematically distorted view of their body weight, was "discovered" by Sir William Gull, who described the condition in 1868 in a lecture at Oxford University. The symptoms have been much debated. Did the condition exist before Gull discovered it? In the 1880s, Jean-Martin Charcot and Sigmund Freud described the anorexic condition as an aspect of hysteria. Although Charcot had demonstrated that hysteria was not an exclusively female condition, the manifestation of anorexia was common in young women and was thought to be associated with the onset of menstruation. More recent research has suggested that anorexia is part of a broader "dietary chaos syndrome." Writers have also argued that the condition is increasingly manifest in young men and that general practitioners have underestimated the prevalence of eating disorders in men. Feminist writers have suggested that the condition is not psychological or behavioral but a social label that describes the complexities of the roles of young women in society (Lorber and Moore 2002). Medical historians have been skeptical about the emergence of the condition in the 1860s, observing that medieval female saints exhibited the syndrome and that self-starvation was part of the ascetic discipline of religious institutions in European Christianity (Brumberg 1988; Bynum 1991).

We can see immediately that a condition that appeared to be distinct and discrete—a false body image resulting in obsessive attitudes toward weight control—is in fact controversial, problematic, and indeterminate. What looked like a set of psychological facts—significant weight loss, disturbed body image, and the onset of symptoms in young women between fifteen and twenty-five years, including amenorrhea, bingeing, and vomiting—turns out to be an interpretation of a wide range of contradictory symptoms. Has anorexia been discovered, or is the discovery a cultural interpretation? Power is central to this controversy because power is the capacity to have one's interpretation treated as authoritative and definitive.

One objection to the preceding example is that psychological conditions such as anorexia, bulimia, and hysteria are inherently fuzzy, but there are some conditions, such as heart disease, to which the constructionist argument does not apply. One can represent heart disease by X-rays, photographs, and anatomical pictures. Heart disease is a fact that is not open to dispute. Here again medical historians might argue that there are many ways to represent and interpret the human body and that anatomical maps are variable (Armstrong 1983). Historians of science argue that we can understand science only as it is practiced in laboratories, clinics, and experimental institutes and that what we might call bench science turns out to be as much conditioned by social and cultural factors as were medieval discussions about the existence of angels. How does culture shape the ways in which we see the body? Medical attempts to distinguish between male and female bodies and between different reproductive functions have been, and continue to be, profoundly influenced by prevailing cultural attitudes toward the social roles of men and women in society (Laqueur 1990).

Constructionism, the idea that things are not discovered but socially produced, is a philosophical perspective that has been applied within both the natural and the social sciences (Hacking 1999). In fact, it has been applied to a great diversity of topics: mathematics, medical conditions, physical objects, and human behavior generally. Everything from serial killers (Jenkins 1994) to "housing facts" (Kemeny 1984) may be socially constructed. In one sense, social constructionism is sociology, because sociologists argue that what appears to be a naturally occurring state of affairs is in fact a product of social relationships or indeed is a social relationship. Constructionism invites us to assume that all facts are necessarily social facts in the sense that social communities produce them. Thus, the professional network of doctors, scientists, and medical researchers is a social community that constructs reality according to its own culture. As a result, medical facts have a history and change over time (Jordanova 1995). Anatomical maps of the human body change for the same reason that maps of the ocean change. William Harvey's discovery of the functions of the heart was published in 1653 as *On Motion of the Heart,* but it was as much a political as a medical treatise on the proper functions of monarchy, as the dedication to King Charles I indicates. It appears, then, that medical knowledge, like political knowledge, is governed by the norms of rhetoric (Erickson

1997). In contemporary sociology, the notion of social constructionism has become influential as a theoretical orientation because developments in the theory of language ("the linguistic turn") have forced social scientists to reassess the legacy of what we might call naturalistic empiricism.

Epistemology is the theory of knowledge. It tells us what we can know with what degree of confidence. Empiricism argues that our senses are our best guide to what exists and can be known. Since no one whose judgment we trust has ever seen a unicorn, we are pretty suspicious of claims that unicorns are alive and well. Naturalistic empiricism claims that our senses are our best guide to knowledge about nature. It claims that, for example, an extreme pain radiating from my upper abdomen to my back and right shoulder is reliable evidence of, or consistent with, having a gall stone stuck in my bile duct. My senses tell me the pain is real and not just a fiction.

Social constructionism raises serious doubts about the reliability of such evidence of the senses, claiming that culture determines how we see and experience the world; that is, our interpretations of evidence are shaped by cultural assumptions. Constructionism draws our attention to how people describe events and experiences by constructing narrative accounts of their encounters with reality. In a recent visit to my local hospital, surgeons examined me to see whether my pancreas was damaged by an infection. Having drawn fluid from around my pancreas, one surgeon told me that there was no evidence of pathology. I exclaimed, "That's good news." Having thought for a while about my observation, the surgeon replied, "There is no such thing as good news; there is only interpretation." The surgeon was making the point that, among other things, my hasty comment on good news had illegitimately gone beyond the evidence of my senses. We might say that the surgeon was, in epistemological terms, a social constructionist rather than a natural empiricist. Nature does not distinguish between pathological fluids and nonpathological fluids. Only human beings employ interpretations to come to such meaningful conclusions. In trying to illustrate this point through a personal experience, I have employed a narrative of my visit to a hospital and my interaction with medical experts. We can readily understand the surgeon's response because I have constructed a story of the events. The notion that social reality is a "narrative text" has become a powerful and persuasive paradigm in sociology and has changed the conventional methodologies of social inquiry.

The debate about the construction of social reality has had an overriding significance in sociological approaches to the human body. For example, it is commonly said that in contemporary society the body has become a project (Shilling 1993). In a modern consumer society, young men may spend a lot of time on bodybuilding exercises. In this sense, men are literally constructing their bodies.

In societies where there is a significant emphasis on youthfulness as a measure of value and beauty, there is considerable emphasis on the physical construction of the body. In particular, the face is an immediate measure of our status in the social hierarchy. We crave above all to be told that we don't look our age. Modern medicine conspires with contemporary consumerism to produce the illusion of endless youthfulness. In this sense, we have to construct our bodies in order to conform socially. The social as opposed to the naturalistic conception of the body has been important in the recent development of medical sociology. For example, the idea that the human body is a cultural object has been analytically important in the sociological criticism of "medical dominance" (Turner 1995a). In this exposition, however, a critical review of social constructionism is undertaken with reference to a range of intellectual problems that surface in an acute form in medical sociology. In this discussion, I do not directly address technical problems in the philosophy of deconstruction, and I am not centrally concerned with narrowly defined matters of epistemology or the philosophy of social science. My research agenda has been to provide medical sociology with a productive base in social theory and, in particular, to connect medical sociology to the sociology of the body.

PRELIMINARY CRITICISM AND ARGUMENT

While being cognizant of the power of the constructionist position in sociology, in this chapter I examine three fundamental criticisms of social constructionism.

First, it is a mistake to assume that social constructionism represents a single or more or less uniform doctrine. There are in fact a great variety of different and contradictory constructionist perspectives. These different types of constructionism present very different accounts of human agency and thus have different implications for an understanding of the relationship between patients, doctors, and disease entities. In this chapter, I shall explore a number of versions of constructionism and examine their contributions to medical sociology.

Second, it is commonly assumed, at least implicitly, that an attack on constructionism—that is, on the notion that medical facts have a history and are variable—results in "essentialism," the notion that there is an unchanging essence about factual reality. We are forced into a false dichotomy between social constructionism and essentialism. These problems are especially difficult in the debate about the social construction of the body. My approach to the issue is to argue that cultural representations of the body are historical, but there is also an experience of embodiment that can be understood only by looking at the body as a social process. The body is a phenomenon that is shaped and cultivated by training and education through our life cycle. It is constantly refined and polished by grooming, toilet practices, diet, and exercise. Social conventions demand that the body be presented in an acceptable fashion. The body is constantly produced through such activities.

It is useful, therefore, for sociology to distinguish between the construction of the body and the phenomenology of embodiment. This distinction is particularly important in medical sociology because it allows the researcher to take a critical stance with respect to the official history of disease and disability and to engage with the subjective experience of illness in terms of the vulnerability of the patient. For example, "the disabled body" might involve an analysis of the rise of the "disability business" (Albrecht 1992) and the political and economic role of stigmatic labels, but "the embodiment of impairment" invokes a different research activity, namely, the study of the everyday world of those with impairment. To take another example, we might say that diabetes is socially constructed because it covers a wide spectrum of symptoms and different types of diabetes have significantly different consequences for patients. Type 2 diabetes is common among people over sixty-five years of age, but it often goes undetected because patients are not aware of the symptoms. For sociological research, it can be useful to distinguish between the social construction of diabetes as a medical category and the everyday experiences of the diabetic. In short, it may be valuable to distinguish between having diabetes as a medical condition and being diabetic as a social role. The former happens to us; the latter is somebody we become.

A third criticism is that constructionism as a cultural theory does not provide convincing answers to important research questions in medical sociology. For example, one illustration of sociological constructionism is the argument that society is a collection of texts and these texts can be understood as forms of rhetoric. If society is an ensemble of narrative texts, however, are all texts of equal importance, and how can we judge their weight? Furthermore, in medical sociology, are some conditions such as "the hyperactive child," more socially constructed than other conditions, such as "gout"? Of course, social constructionism shares these issues with earlier forms of the sociology of knowledge, namely, the problem of how one measures or understands the social effects of discourses, texts, or statements regarded as ideological, or socially constructed. Theories of ideology (and, by extension, theories of social construction) have not been particularly successful in showing that a pervasive set of beliefs has consistent effects or consequences on belief and practice such that it could be said to constitute a dominant ideology or a dominant discourse (Abercrombie, Hill, and Turner 1980). Without a more robust research methodology, sociological interpretations of social texts have the same force, or lack of it, as literary interpretations, and sociological theory remains largely "decorative" (Rojek and Turner 2000). There is an important sociological difference, for example, between claiming that anorexia is socially constructed and exploring the intended and unintended consequences of anorexia in the lives of individuals. The study of discourse, rhetoric, and ideology does not necessarily produce convincing arguments about social consequences because it treats social consequences as yet another text. In short, social constructionist arguments are often disconcertingly circular.

For some critics, social construction has a shock value because it can be liberating to realize suddenly that something that is stigmatizing—such as a medical condition—is constructed; the troubling condition is not part of the nature of things, people, or human society (Hacking 1999, 35). This liberating aspect of the intellectual challenge of constructionism explains the enduring attraction of Peter Berger's *Invitation to Sociology* (1963), which, among other things, shows how what we take to be the uniqueness of a romantic attachment is merely a social institution. The initial intellectual and political impetus behind constructionism may now be exhausted, however, and as an intellectual position it is not adequate for a number of reasons. Criticism of constructionism indicates that we need a phenomenological understanding of the experiences of embodiment to develop a comprehensive sociology of health and illness. We need good phenomenological answers to such basic questions as, What is it like to be chronically sick? What is it like to be infirm, frail, or old? As I have indicated, constructionism should be properly applied to the body as a classificatory system, but as an analysis of embodiment it is less appropriate as a set of practices and experiences. We need a foundationalist view of embodiment to develop an ethics and politics of the body that can take account of patients' experiences and personal narratives. The notions of the vulnerability of the body and the precariousness of institutions offer powerful metatheoretical assumptions for medical sociology.

Because the constructionist account of medical classification provides a very partial basis for a comprehensive medical sociology, we need to develop a position that integrates the construction of the body as a cultural object and the embodiment of people in the everyday world. This integration is theoretically important for the somewhat conventional argument that sociology, like economics and politics, requires a theory of social action. Action requires agency and an actor, and the human agents of social action and interaction are embodied. Such an interpretation of sociology does not necessarily involve methodological individualism because sociology also presupposes the institutionalization of action. Actions are never wholly random or individual; they are produced by and shaped through institutionalization. In order to develop this sociology of embodiment, actions, and institutions, we need a conception of embodiment rather than simply a theory of the classification of bodies. A constructionist approach to the body and health will not allow us a comprehensive understanding of the emotions that surround pain and suffering in the everyday world of the patient (S. J. Williams 2003).

POLITICS AND SOCIAL CONSTRUCTION

If social constructionism is problematic as an epistemology, why should medical sociology persist with its applications? Are there grounds for simply abandoning the project of social constructionism in medical sociology? There is at least one important reason for maintaining social constructionism: the nature of medical practice itself. Medicine is a discipline that combines both science and art. It relies heavily on biology, chemistry, and physiology to explain the underlying causes of disease; it is increasingly dependent on information science and computerization. Finally, it seeks to cure disease through the application of science to the human body, but it also purports to care for the patient by understanding the meaning of disease. The German philosopher Hans-Georg Gadamer referred to this combination of science and art as "the enigma of health" and claimed that medicine is an "art of healing in a scientific age." As an art, medicine involves diagnosis and interpretation of symptoms in order to establish appropriate care for the patient. Diagnosis involves the doctor in "knowing how to distinguish" between competing interpretations of a range of symptoms that are exhibited by a patient's condition. While scientific data from observational recordings, blood samples, X-rays, and CAT scans play a major part in a doctor's diagnostic decisions, "there still exists, even today, a particularly wide scope for the exercise of doctor's powers of judgement" (1996, 19). An experienced doctor undertaking a diagnosis will recognize that the scientific data are not confirmed facts but evidence that helps the doctor reach an interpretation of the patient's condition. The isolated facts or observational data about a patient make sense (a meaning) only when they are placed in relationship to each other within a diagnostic paradigm; they have meaning only when they are interpreted. They make medical sense only when they are classified within a nosological map (King 1982). We might conclude by saying that medical facts make sense only when they have been constructed by nosology, or the theory of the classification of diseases.

In restoring the patient to health, the doctor has to make judgments about the patient's psychological state and his or her social circumstances. Does the patient have sufficient social support to stay at home, or should the patient be taken into care? Are the patient's injuries the result of domestic violence? In making these judgments about social circumstances, the doctor is working implicitly as an applied sociologist. Such judgments about the patient are sociological because they attempt to make an assessment about issues relating to gender, socioeconomic status, social competence, and social circumstances. Because the doctor is involved in the interpretation of the social life of the patient, he or she is necessarily involved in a social construction of the patient. Thus, social constructions are important for the doctor's diagnostic conclusions about the patient's condition. Without them, the doctor could not make relevant diagnostic judgments, but they are nevertheless constructions. Because these medical judgments are constructions, we need to examine the social conditions that make them persuasive, effective, and legitimate. How does the professional power of doctors function to give their diagnostic interpretations social authority and credibility? Because there is an intimate connection between professional power and social knowledge, these medical constructions are suitable and important topics for sociological research.

Although I criticize constructionism, I recognize that it has been politically important in social movements, for example, the women's movement and feminism, the disability movement, and social conflicts about age and aging (Lorber and

Moore 2002). Political deployments of constructionist theories arise in contexts within which traditional categories of behavior have been challenged and contested. Political confrontation means that conventional patterns of behavior are no longer taken for granted and, hence, their "plausibility structures" are shattered. For example, the idea that anorexia is socially constructed typically arises in a situation where women want to deny the importance of the physiological foundations of sex differences in social behavior—"anatomy is not destiny." The constructionist critique also involves protest against the dominant commercial norms of feminine beauty, which are regarded as problematic for women's health. Constructionism has been important in the political debate about menopause and premenstrual syndrome (Parlee 1994). Menopause is highly contentious because its manifestations are diverse and vary significantly among societies. By contrast, where categories of behavior or disease are not overtly politicized, the question of their social construction tends not to occur. For example, while obesity and anorexia are politically charged, diabetes does not appear to be. Diabetes does not figure into social movements, and there is little evidence of any desire on the part of medical sociologists to deconstruct, question, or criticize diabetes as a medical category. It affects many middle-aged Americans, but there has not been a diabetes lobby to suggest that diabetes is a political condition. Diseases that are not politically contested are assumed to be unfortunate facts of life, not social constructs. By contrast, conditions that are shot through with political struggles are often regarded as social constructs.

Social constructionism is therefore probably best regarded as a historical account of how certain disease or sickness categories become accepted over time by the medical profession or by society and how that historical process is shaped by political struggles and economic interests. The historical reception of such "medical conditions" as premenstrual syndrome, repetitive strain injury, irritable bowel syndrome, and hyperactivity are particularly instructive illustrations of how a nonspecific discomfort or social issue can be transformed over time into a distinctive medical condition as a consequence of the lobbying by the sufferers of the condition. Medical anthropologists have shown how Western medical conditions such as premenstrual syndrome or brain death and technologies such as organ harvesting are often exported to other cultures where they were previously unknown or absent (Lock, Young, and Cambrosio 2000).

GENDER AND THE BODY

The sociology of the body has also been developed in response to questions of patriarchy, gender, sex, and sexuality (Bordo 1993). The question of the gendered nature of power has been facilitated by feminist and gay writing on the body (Richardson 2000; Richardson and Seidman 2002). Much feminist theory about the body has been developed through French social theory, especially by Julia Kristeva, Hélène Cixous, and Luce Irigaray (Pateman and Gross 1986). The specific application of this theoretical tradition to the body has been undertaken by a variety of feminist writers for very different purposes, but there are common features to the logic of the underlying argument. French feminists challenged the view of sexuality in Freud and Jacques Lacan and turned to the body to celebrate female difference. Freud had treated female sexuality as a lack or an absence, which he described in terms of envy of the penis. In opposition to Freud, they defined female sexuality as open, dispersed, and multiple and developed a vision of female "otherness" as a challenge to male power. Kristeva celebrated the ancient conflict between men and women, emphasizing their fundamental psychological and social differences. The notion of female specificity has brought a charge of "essentialism" against this tradition in which men and women in their very essence are different and separate. As a counterweight to the problem of biological determinism, feminist theory, following Kristeva, has emphasized the importance of symbolic power, rather than biological difference, in the creation of the male-female dichotomy. For Kristeva and her followers, the difference between men and women is rooted in culture or symbolic power. The politics of sexual difference has thus established the centrality of the socially constructed body; it also requires the view that alleged emotional and moral differences between men and women (for example, women are more caring and sensitive than men) are also social products and therefore can be changed and transformed. The pioneering work of anthropologists like Margaret Mead was effective in demonstrating, for example, that what we take to be the fixed emotional attributes of men and women, such as aggression or caring, are in fact features of socialization in different social roles in different cultures. While there is a social division of gender activities, those roles and status positions have no necessary or determinate relationship to biological sex. Although Mead did not refer to her cultural anthropology as constructionist, *Sex and Temperament in Three Primitive Societies* (1935) and other publications had a major impact on early feminist criticism of conventional views of the "natural" divisions between men and women.

Recent feminist literature has rejected the essentialism of traditional social science approaches to sexual identity and sexuality. Thus, sexuality has a history, being constructed by the powerful discourses of religion, medicine, and law. One objection to this form of social constructionism might be that while social roles are constructed, anatomy is not. Whatever the role of culture in shaping personality, men and women just have different bodies. Recent historical writing on the history of anatomy is instructive in this context. For example, medieval theories of sexuality upheld the doctrine of a single sex with dichotomous genders. The female body was simply a weakened, deformed, or inverted form of the male body (Laqueur 1990). Anatomical investigation was unable to transform this rigid ideological notion into an alternative discourse until the emergence of Freudian psychoanalysis. A considerable amount of contemporary scholarship, therefore, has gone into the historical analysis of the impact of Christian ideology on the presentation of gender differences as differences of a moral order (Ariès and Béjin 1985; Rousselle 1988). The Enlightenment, which in many areas of social life attempted to overturn traditional assumptions, held that women were determined by their reproductive functions, and the role of Enlightenment medicine was to understand scientifically the natural differentiation between men and women (Steinbrugge 1995). Although much of this analysis is concerned with the historical shaping of the difference between men and women, gender differences continue to play a major role in the representation of power and authority in contemporary industrial societies. For example, Emily Martin, in *The Women in the Body* (1987), has presented a fascinating analysis of the relationship between industrial production and reproduction in which, for example, the reproduction of children is still referred to as labor.

One controversial issue in the feminist critique of contemporary medical science is menopause. From the standpoint of social constructionism, menopause has been medicalized and treated as a health risk for which there are medical solutions and therapies, such as hormone replacement therapy (HRT). Menopause has in fact been constructed as a disease of estrogen deficiency, and the medical model presents an overwhelmingly negative view of the process in terms of both psychological and physical disturbance. Although there has been an important growth of self-help literature, the literature is dominated by biomedical accounts (Lyons and Griffin 2003). In clinical encounters, where popular or lay views of menopause are necessarily treated as unreliable, the doctor's view of the benefits of HRT will dominate the transaction between patient and doctor (Masse and Legare 2001). By contrast, feminist research argues that menopause should not be taken out of its social context and should be regarded as part of a "status passage" to midlife that involves many social as well as biological changes (Ballard, Kuh, and Wadsworth 2001). By treating menopause as a socially constructed condition, women have been able to develop alternative and positive views of it, but the biomedical model is often dominant in medical settings, where the pharmaceutical companies have a clear commercial interest in HRT and related therapies (Parlee 1994).

Although constructionism has been an important component of feminist debates about women's health, there has been a growing awareness of men's health. Radical changes in explanations of men's health over time suggest that these health issues are subject to changes in public attitudes toward health, work, and gender (Arber 1997). Men's health is also constructed by changes in health perceptions that are influenced by diagnostic fashions. One illustration is the notion of "executive disease" that emerged in the 1950s to explain the high prevalence of coronary heart disease among middle-class white-collar men in American corporate culture (Riska 2002). The high levels of stress that were associated with business culture produced what was known in popular terminology as hurry sickness, but a technical term from the medical diagnosis by American cardiologists emerged in 1959 to explain the prevalence of the problem: type-A men. According to Meyer Friedman and Ray Rosenman (1959), type-A men are competitive and ambitious and live with an inescapable sense of urgency. Their attitudes are accompanied in behavioral terms by rapid body movements, tense facial musculature, teeth clenching, and unconscious gesturing. These ambitious and competitive men were required by the new economic and management environment of postwar America, and this new stratum of white-collar employees became the topic of sociological study. In *The Organization Man,* W. H. Whyte (1956) showed how the corporation demanded total commitment and expected its executives to move from town to town or from country to country in meeting organizational goals. The successful organization man was a spiralist moving upward through various positions in the company, but the social costs of a spiralist career were high: the absence of any roots in the community, few lasting friendships, and high divorce rates. The health costs of spiraling ambition were also high for type-A men: stress and heart disease.

In the late 1970s and 1980s, the type-A man slowly disappeared as a popular diagnostic category and was replaced by the idea of "the hardy executive" (Maddi and Kobasa 1984). As a psychological disposition, "hardiness" protected executives from the negative health consequences of stress. The hardy executive has control over his life, is committed to his work, and regards stressful situations as a creative challenge. Whereas the type-A man suffered from powerlessness and alienation, the hardy executive develops a positive attitude to promotion and job change. Hardiness gradually acquired recognition in the medical literature as a psychological factor that is important in health protection.

While type-A man and the hardy executive as concepts have been criticized in the professional medical literature, they are useful indicators of changing public attitudes toward health. The type-A man flourished in a 1950s business world that had not developed a corporate culture of physical fitness. By contrast, modern corporations are aware of the dangers of stress and isolation for the health of their employees. The hardy executive reflects a corporate culture that takes diet and exercise seriously but also emphasizes personal responsibility for health, encouraging executives to embrace healthy lifestyles. The result is that rates of coronary heart disease have declined significantly in the American professional middle classes (Riska 2002, 354). These diagnostic labels—type-A man and hardy executive—are social constructs that reflect real changes in heart disease and the health consciousness of men in professional status groups.

Both menopause and the stressful life of type-A man are related to stages in the life cycle. In modern society, aging is contested because there are no clear agreements about the nature of aging in relation to lifestyle. Because aging is politically contested, arguments emerge to suggest that it is constructed. Menopause, in particular, has become a critical political issue because it raises questions about the proper role or roles of women in society.

SOCIOLOGICAL CONSTRUCTIONISM

Peter Berger and Thomas Luckmann's *Social Construction of Reality* (1966) can be regarded as the classical text of social constructionism in sociology. Berger's general sociology has been influenced by the philosophical anthropology of Arnold Gehlen (1980, 1988); Berger has been explicit about the importance of Gehlen's philosophical anthropology in the development of his own work (Berger and Kellner 1965). Gehlen argued that human beings are "not yet finished animals." By this notion, he meant that human beings are, in biological terms, not fully equipped to deal with the world into which they are involuntarily inserted. They have no finite instinctual basis that is specific to a given environment, and they depend on a long period of socialization in order to adapt to the world. In order to cope with the openness of their world, human beings have to create a cultural dimension to replace or supplement their instinctual environment. It is this biological incompleteness that provides an anthropological explanation for the origin of human social institutions.

Berger and Luckmann (1966) adopted Gehlen's position to argue that since human beings are biologically underdeveloped, they have to construct a "social canopy" around themselves in order to complete or supplement their biology. Social institutions are the bridges between humans and their physical environment, and it is through these institutions that human life becomes coherent, meaningful, and continuous. In filling the gap created by instinctual deprivation, institutions provide humans with relief from the tensions generated by undirected instinctual drives. Over time, institutions are taken for granted and become an aspect of the background of social action. The foreground is occupied by reflexive, practical, and conscious activities. With modernization, there is a process of deinstitutionalization, with the result that the background becomes less reliable, more open to negotiation, culturally thinner, and increasingly an object of reflection. Accordingly, the foreground expands, and life is seen to be risky and reflexive. The objective and sacred institutions of the past recede, and modern life becomes subjective, contingent, and uncertain. In fact, we live in a world of secondary or quasi institutions.

These institutions require a stable "plausibility structure," of which sociology offers a basic but far-reaching criticism (Berger 1963). Institutions, which we take for granted and regard as natural, are shown to be socially constructed and precarious. We become disillusioned with these "social facts" because we can see that they are human products. Berger also shows, however, that while they are constructed, they are socially necessary, and collective life would be intolerable without them. Indeed, Berger's constructivist critique suggests that we would be wise to discard our sociological awareness that, for example, identity, marriage, and honor are socially constructed, because their legitimacy and effectiveness depend on their taken-for-granted facticity. Similarly, the doctor-patient relationship requires a taken-for-granted trust that can be disrupted by sociological research into its precariousness.

Berger's version of social constructionism has become unfashionable because it is not easily reconciled—for example, with the radical deconstruction of sexual categories by feminist theory, the attack on racial identities by subaltern studies, or the rejection of determined and fixed homosexual identities by queer theory. In short, popular forms of social constructionism are basically antiessentialist, whereas Berger's sociology is rooted in a foundationalist epistemology that recognizes the need for social order and cultural stability if the world is to have any meaning. Because Berger deconstructs identity from an interpretation of the biological characteristics of human beings, their instinctual incompleteness, his work conflicts with the contemporary tendency of constructionism to reject biological explanations of human nature and social institutions. Modern constructionism emphasizes, in contrast to Berger's theory, the fluidity of identity. Despite the ironic nature of Berger and Luckmann's sociology of knowledge, their position is deterministic in the sense that society cannot exist without functional plausibility structures. To them, the sacred canopy, to be sacred, must exist in society as a social fact. Berger's constructionism ultimately retreats from political radicalism in the interests of social cohesion (Berger 1998) because the sacred canopy must remain in place if disorder and anomie are to be avoided.

Berger's sociology has had importance for the development of sociology in general, but his analysis of knowledge has had a more direct impact on the sociology of religion than on medical sociology. In recent years, Michel Foucault's treatment of knowledge and power has been influential in sociology as a whole, but Foucault has had a specific relevance for medical sociology. For Foucault, knowledge is always connected to—rather than separated from—power, and medical knowledge provides doctors with a special mechanism of power.

MICHEL FOUCAULT AND THE DISCOURSE OF THE BODY

Foucault has made a significant contribution to the development of a strand of social science that has been labeled post-structuralism. In retrospect, it is now clear that Foucault made two specific contributions to contemporary social science: an analysis of power and a contribution to the understanding of the emergence of the modern self through various educational technologies. Foucault's analysis of power has proved particularly useful in understanding the functions of the medical profession and the clinic (1973, 1980b). His theory of power was a critical reaction to both French Marxism and the existentialism of Jean-Paul Sartre. He attempted to challenge the Marxist conceptualization of power as a macro structure—such as the state—that functions to support capitalism and is displayed through major public institutions, such as the police, law, and state agencies. Foucault saw power as a relationship that was localized, dispersed, and diffused through the social system, operating at a micro or covert level through sets of specific practices. Power is embodied in the day-to-day practices of the medical profession within the clinic, the activities of social workers, the daily decision making of legal officers, and the religious practices of the church via the confessional. This view of power is closely associated with Foucault's fascination with discipline—namely, the idea that power comes to exist by means of the disciplinary practices that produce particular individuals, institutions, and cultural arrangements. He became particularly interested in the social theories of the English philosopher Jeremy Bentham, who in the nineteenth century rejected physical punishment as a method of controlling criminals and set about changing the architectural design of prisons to reflect his view that prisons should be useful rather than punitive. His design of prisons, called a panopticon, was intended to maximize the surveillance of prison inmates. Bentham's plan of the panopticon was an architectural model of total surveillance that also provided guidelines for the construction of schools and hospitals, in which children and patients could be regulated economically and efficiently.

The disciplinary management of society results in a "carceral," a form of society in which Bentham's principles of the panopticon are institutionalized in society through everyday arrangements. These ideas about power were further elaborated by Foucault's interest in governmentality—a system of power that articulates the triangular relationship between sovereignty, discipline, and government (1991). Governmentality emerged in the eighteenth century as a mechanism for regulating and controlling populations through an apparatus of security. This governmental apparatus required a whole series of specific *savoirs* (knowledges) and was the foundation for the rise of the administrative state.

A further important feature of Foucault's work was the analysis of the relationship between power and knowledge. Whereas liberal theory tended to separate power and knowledge on the grounds that truth is always corrupted by the exercise of power, Foucault saw that power and knowledge are always inevitably and inextricably interconnected. Any extension of power involves an increase in knowledge, and every elaboration of knowledge involves an increase in power. Foucault typically approached this question through a consideration of populations and bodies. For example, the growth of penology and criminology was closely associated with the development of panoptic principles of surveillance and control. In a similar fashion, he saw the whole development of psychology and psychiatry in terms of forms of knowledge and an extension of power over the subordinate populations of urban Europe. Foucault's *Order of Things* (1970) showed the intimate relationships between forms of surveillance and control and the development of social scientific knowledge. In fact, Foucault normally spoke about knowledge in the plural in order to illustrate the notion that specific forms of power require highly specific and detailed formations of knowledge. Foucault's conceptual apparatus, built around the study of the history of ideas, the analysis of power, and the explication of forms of discipline, proved enormously useful and important for medical sociologists in their attempt to understand the forms of power assumed by medical practices. Foucault's work permitted sociologists to think about the medicalization of society within a new framework, where the exercise of medical power was seen in terms of local, diffuse practices. The medical sociology inspired by Foucault is heavily informed by theoretical and philosophical analysis of self, discipline, and sexuality; it is highly critical of established psychiatry and clinical medicine, seeking to provide alternative ways of examining mental illness and disease; it places power and knowledge at the center of the sociological understanding of medical institutions; and it shows how medical ideas of the moral character of disease operate at an everyday level. His perspective has been employed to understand such diverse topics as the regulation of the elderly (Katz 1996), the meaning of surgery (N. J. Fox 1992), the power of medical professions (Turner 1995a), and the anatomy lesson (Armstrong 1983).

For Foucault, the study of medicine is part of a larger intellectual program, one that examines the evolution of sexuality and the self in European societies from classical Greece through early Christianity to modern times and the way that evolution was intimately bound up with the transformation of medicine (Foucault 1985, 1986). In his final publications, Foucault appeared to turn more and more to an analysis of the self in the context of medical history and the development of sexuality. His interest in how the self in Western societies was an effect of discourse and disciplines of the self became increasingly obvious in his studies of "technologies of the self" (L. H. Martin, Gutman, and Hutton 1988). Medicine replaced religion as the basis of the construction of ethics and the self in modern society.

For Foucault, the body is the crucial topic in the evolution of these regulative practices. The normalization of the body is the outcome of new forms of knowledge and surveillance associated with the control of captive populations, such as armies, prisoners, and the mentally ill. The body is the focus of military disciplinary practices, but it is also subject to the monastic regulation of medieval Catholicism. The Foucauldian critique of modern medicine is that it represents a form of government that controls individual transgression through a network of local normative constraints. It is an effective, localized institution of normative coercion meant to produce compliant patients. Medicine involves a government of the body (Turner 1992). Although there was significant evolution and change in Foucault's social philosophy, it is clear that the body and populations played a major role in the analytic structure of his work.

TECHNOLOGY AND THE BODY

The idea that the body can be easily or endlessly transformed by technology is a modern utopian idea. I refer critically to this position as utopian because it converts reality into a fiction in which anything in principle is technologically possible. It is the utopian side of the dystopian, or Frankenstein, view of gender, science, and the human body. Technological utopianism celebrates or promotes a "mirage of health" (Dubos 1960). In this model, the traditional afflictions of humanity could be removed by science, the earth could be made more abundant, and heart conditions, strokes, and cancer could be eliminated. Genetic counseling, artificial reproduction, genetic engineering, and cloning are in many senses spectacular illustrations of the possibilities opened up by the new genetics. These scientific developments are forging a new imagination for constructing genetic maps of human life (Rothman 1998). They thus suggest a special meaning for constructionism that is close to social engineering through the application of genetic science. And they present society or, more specifically, governments with an opportunity for political and social control through a modern eugenics. My argument in this section, however, is that these technological transformations of the human body do not bring about the disappearance of the body, and this argument remains a pressing issue for governments in modern society.

The development of modern technology provides the potential to replace bodily functions and organs and to repair and upgrade the performance of the human body. It can do this in two ways. First, by directly altering the infrastructure of the body, genetic engineering represents a further step in a series of increasingly radical techniques that will produce a society of "posthumans." By posthuman, Francis Fukuyama (2002) means that scientific transformations of the human body—for example, by cloning—may be so profound that we will no longer be able to refer to ourselves meaningfully as human. Second, by constructing artificial devices and altering the immediate near-to-body environment, technology can augment and replace human capacities through systems designed to increase empowerment. These technologies are now often simple devices, such as wheelchairs, ventilators, prostheses, and voice synthesizers, but they may include computers as well. The possibility that information science, computers, and biology may combine to change the human body has led to speculation about cyborgs and techno-persons. In the former case, the inner structure of the body is changed or redesigned with technological replacement parts or devices, and in the latter case the body is fitted into a new "outer skin" of specially designed devices, machines, and technological environments.

There has been considerable interest in the social implications of machine-body fusions, or cyborgs. For example, there has long been a strong association between technology and masculinity. In popular culture, *RoboCop* was at one stage the ultimate cyborg, the merging of machine and organism, but the character also incorporated traditional gender themes of power and sexuality. The technology of *RoboCop* now looks antiquated by comparison with the computerized world of *The Terminator, Star Wars,* and *The Matrix.* The *homo faber* perspective remains a vivid myth, however, that conceptualizes man as the maker and builder, whose hands are potent tools. This pervasive modern myth elevates a particular form of masculinity and denies the potential of alternative relations between the body and technology. In recent years, however, feminists have begun to confront the relationship between women and technology and to explore the potential benefits that not only reproductive technologies but also the reproductive and emancipatory implications of new forms of technology will have for women (Haraway 1991).

The new information technology and the potential of virtual reality and cyberspace attracted great interest. Computer simulations and networks create the possibilities of new experiences of disembodiment, reembodiment, and emotional attachment. All of these phenomena threaten to transform conventional assumptions about the nature of social relationships.

Technological construction, as an implicit framework, can also be said to include the political statements of performance artists like Stelarc and Orlan. Stelarc has, through a series of artistic performances, explored the interconnections between the body, technology, and the environment to promote the idea of the end of the body as a natural phenomenon (Fleming 2002). In the case of Orlan, the surgical reconstructions of her face are intended to be performances in which she ironically calls into question the transformation of women's bodies by cosmetics and cosmetic surgery. By transforming surgery into a public drama, she critically explores the exploitative relationships between cosmetics, medical practice, and gender stereotypes. She is literally showing that medical technology can socially reconstruct her body. Here we see the body being used as a site on which occurs a performance that delivers a powerful political statement (Featherstone 2000). Although this technological dimension is an underdeveloped aspect of social constructionism, I include it here in contrast to more deterministic models of the cultural production of the body. Orlan's surgery ironically displays the power of medical technology while also calling technology into question as part of the commercial apparatus of a consumer society.

Cosmetic surgery involves the actual reconstruction of the "natural" body in order to produce social—that is, aesthetic—effects. According to the British Association of Aesthetic Plastic Surgeons, there are no official statistics in the United Kingdom for the number of women having cosmetic surgery, but it is estimated that in 2000 there were seventy-two thousand surgical procedures. The "industry" is worth about £150 million ($250 million) per annum. The most common procedures for women are breast and facial surgery. In the United States, the cosmetic industry is clearly much larger and more acceptable. In 1998, there were 2.8 million cosmetic surgical procedures, of which 10 percent were performed on men (K. Davis 1995, 2002). While aesthetic surgery is becoming routine, the negative effects of cosmetic surgery have come to public attention through sensational cases, such as the death of Lolo Ferrari, whose eighteen operations created what were reputed to be the largest breasts in the world, a 54G cup. There are other celebrity cases, such as Jocelyne Wildenstein, who has shaped her face in the image of a leopard (Pitts 2003). Orlan's surgical performances are designed to bring into question the alliance between medicine, market, and aesthetics in a consumer society where the human (typically female) body is being simultaneously physically and socially reconstructed. With the graying of the population, we can expect that, given the emphasis on youth and beauty in American society, cosmetic surgery will become almost as routine and commonplace as a visit to the dentist.

If the body is socially constructed, some theorists of postmodern cyborgs suggest, then the body with its narratives or inscriptions of sex and gender is disappearing with the rise of the techno-body. For postmodern theorists of extreme or hyper modernity (Kroker and Kroker 1987), the natural body has no ontological status and has been deconstructed by a series of invasions to produce the "panic body." Panic bodies are merely "inscribed surfaces" that function as the conduits of the debris of technological civilization. This postmodern analysis of the impact of hypermodernity on the body is rhetorically provocative (Balsam 1995), but it is a remarkably limited view of the body in society. It does not touch on the economic aspect of the way bodies in modern medicine might be reconstructed, namely, through the exchange of organs. The global market in body "spare parts" should alert us to profound differences in the place of the body in rich and poor societies. The sale of organs and the gross inequalities in the organ marketplace conjure up a radically different picture of the "disappearance of the body." The postmodern body belongs to the utopian vision of the disappearing body because it provides little conceptual space for not only death and violence in the third world (Scheper-Hughes 1992) but also the routine problems of aging and decay in the everyday world of rich societies (Riggs and Turner 1999).

This technological perspective on the body is utopian in one additional sense: it pays little attention to the alienation and exploitation of the body by a consumer-driven technological society. Far from disappearing, the body in a "cool" technological society becomes increasingly obtrusive because its structures and rhythms do not always easily fit the demands of a machine age. It appears likely that the emergence of repetitive strain injury among office workers in the 1980s was a consequence of the rapid introduction of computers into white-collar and professional occupations. We are yet to understand fully the long-term impact of computers, mobile phones, or microwaves on health. The emergence of "acoustic shock" in commercial telephone call centers is another illustration of the tensions between the body and technology. The transformation or reconstruction of the body in hypermodernity by means of advanced technology does not indicate its disappearance (Turner 2001a). It is the vulnerability of the body with respect to technology that is important.

HUMAN VULNERABILITY

I have presented a variety of arguments about the social construction of knowledge and, hence, the social construction of medical knowledge. These arguments are important and reflect major sociological contributions to understanding social reality. I want now, however, to present an alternative position, one based on the idea of human vulnerability and the precariousness of social institutions. This alternative does not wholly reject constructionism but argues that constructionism is limited. The basic argument is that human beings are ontologically vulnerable and the natural environment uncertain. In order to protect themselves from the vagaries or afflictions of existence, people must build social institutions, especially political, familial, and ecclesiastical institutions that come to constitute what we call society. We need the companionship of other people in society to provide us with the means of mutual support, and we need the comfort of social institutions as the means of fortifying our existence. These institutions are themselves precarious, however, and cannot provide an entirely reliable social environment. This common vulnerability creates social patterns of dependency and connectedness because we cannot satisfy our needs in isolation (Turner 1997a). While the human body is socially constructed in the sense that it is always open to interpretation, there are basic aspects of human life that are not wholly context dependent. Our vulnerability is variable, but all humans, by virtue of their common humanity, are vulnerable.

The concept of vulnerability is derived from the Latin *vulnus,* or "wound." It is instructive from my perspective that vulnerability should have such an obviously corporeal origin. The historical etymology of the word shows us that in the seventeenth century *vulnerability* had both a passive and an active significance, namely, "to be wounded" and "to wound." *To vulnerate* is "to wound," but in its modern usage it has become a passive state, "to be wounded." In its modern form, *vulnerability* has also become more abstract: it refers to human exposure to psychological or moral damage. It refers increasingly to our capacity to suffer morally and spiritually rather than to our physical exposure to pain. This openness to wounding is part of what Berger (1980) has called our "world openness," namely, that we do not live in a biologically determined or species-specific environment that is secure. To be vulnerable as a human being is to possess a structure of sentiments, feelings, and emotions by which we can steer a passage through the social order (Barbalet 1998; Turner 2000b).

We are vulnerable because we are embodied. I propose to treat embodiment not as a static entity but as a series of social processes taking place in the life course. Embodiment is a life process that requires the learning of body techniques such as walking, sitting, dancing, and eating. It is the ensemble of such corporal practices, which produce and give a body its place in everyday life. Embodiment locates, or places, particular bodies within a social habitus. It involves the production of a sensuous and practical presence in the life world (Turner 1997b, 1999a). Embodiment is our lived experience of the sensual body, and the meaning of embodiment can be derived from Karl Marx's idea of praxis (1964) or from Pierre Bourdieu's notions of practice and habitus (1990). It concerns the various ways in which we actively shape the everyday world. An individual's embodiment is not an isolated project; it is located within a social world of interconnected social actors. While it is the process of making and becoming a body, it is also the project of making a self. Embodiment and self-creation are mutually dependent and self-reinforcing projects because I am recognized as a separate and specific individual through my embodiment. Embodiment is the mode by which human beings practically engage with and apprehend the world.

While human beings are vulnerable, they also live in a social world that is precarious. Social and political precariousness includes the inability of political institutions to protect and serve the interests of individuals, the failure of social institutions to cope with social change, the inability of social institutions to reconcile the conflict of collective and individual interests, and finally the social problems of coping with generational exchanges in terms of equity. Institutions have to be built up over time and often fail to respond quickly to social change. The process of institutionalization tends to be conservative and cannot address the changing aspirations of new generations. Institutional precariousness is not a special aspect of modern society. The transformations of religious charisma, such as prophecy, into tradition were familiar aspects of premodern societies. In the modern economy, organizational failures through takeovers, mergers, corporate corruption, organizational stress, inflation, and globalization are permanent features of the restructuring of the business world. Business failures are a daily feature of the modern economy. On a larger canvas, global instability has resulted from the collapse of the Soviet Union and Communist regimes as a consequence of the inability of rigid bureaucratic systems and privileged elites to respond to economic and social strain. Illustrations of institutional precariousness abound, and modern social systems are incapable of resolving their system complexities. Instability is a ubiquitous feature of human society, but social precariousness appears to be a particular problem of modernity.

While the notion of vulnerability might suggest an individualistic approach, the notion of interconnectedness indicates that human beings are always and already social. We are deeply involved socially through language and socialization. Technological and medical changes threaten this interconnectedness of the social world, however. Television has converted many young people into couch potatoes whose social connections with the world outside the home are minimal. The speed of modern life has made us dependent on fast food, snacks, ready-made meals, the microwave, and takeout from McDonald's. The result is that the social bonding that came with the family meal, the Sunday roast, and the prepared breakfast has eroded. Medical technology may make traditional parenting through heterosexual intercourse unnecessary. Medicine would thereby transform our relationship to "our" offspring and transform the traditional family as well. This scenario is implied in Fukuyama's notion of posthumans. Cyborgs and other technologies may transform the nature of embodiment and remove this interconnectedness of human life. Can there be a traditional social world when technology has transformed the conditions of our own embodiment? Will advances in medical technology make us less vulnerable? Can social engineering make our human world less precarious?

There are, consequently, two important objections to the notions of the vulnerability of the body and the precariousness of institutions that we must consider. From a medical point of view, one might argue that medical developments such as the vaccination have made us less vulnerable, and we can measure these improvements by means of simple data on mortality rates and life expectancy. The second point of view might be that institutions are not necessarily precarious and that medical institutions such as the hospital are illustrations of robust institutionalization. The counterarguments would be that because we live longer, we are subject to increasing rates of morbidity in old age. We live longer but with higher rates of dependency and disability. Hospitals provide excellent services to their patients, and antiseptics have played a major role in the transformation of surgery, but hospitals remain dangerous environments where secondary infections can have troublesome consequences. Hospitals are precarious institutions because the more they rely on advanced technology to provide surgical responses to disease and disability, the greater the risk of unintended consequences.

The real argument in support of the interrelated concepts of vulnerability and precariousness is their connection to social capital. If Robert Putnam's arguments about bowling alone are correct, then the United States is moving toward a society of low participation in civil society, increasing isolation of the elderly, and declining social interconnectedness. Vulnerable groups in society—the elderly, the impaired, the unemployed, and the uninsured—are disconnected from civil society. Social capital can be regarded as a collective fund that offsets the vulnerability we experience as individuals and the precariousness of public institutions. The intermediate associations that Durkheim regarded as counterweights to the negative impact of individualism and anomie are weak, and hence isolated individuals are exposed to negative social currents. The social interconnectedness that results from human dependency in the life course is in decline as a consequence of the erosion and depletion of social capital.

CONCLUSION: CLASSIFICATION, DISEASE,
AND THE QUIDDITY OF LIFE

Although from a sociological point of view constructionist arguments are persuasive, they present in many respects a limited view of scientific beliefs. A critic might argue that while lay beliefs and everyday assumptions about health and illness are indeed the products of the everyday experiences of being sick, the clinical categories of disease, which arise from close scientific inspection and doctors' observations of symptoms, are not socially constructed and do not change significantly over time. One version of this argument would be to claim that some concepts of disease are more socially constructed than others (Turner 1992, 106). What people say or believe about a disease changes over time, but the clinical condition itself is relatively consistent. For example, Hippocrates' clinical description of mumps could easily be identified and confirmed by a contemporary general practitioner. Ilza Veith (1981, 222) argues that "what is unchanged is disease. What did change, however, is the way in which disease was looked upon." Lester King (1982, 149), who made a useful distinction between a clinical entity and a disease entity, facilitated our understanding of this contrast. A clinical entity (from *klinē*, or "bed") is a configuration, or pattern, that is observed by a doctor in a bed-side interaction with a patient. The concept is thus closely linked to the practice of medicine. A disease entity is knowledge about a condition. Doctors' observations, statistical information, and laboratory tests produce this knowledge. As a disease entity becomes scientifically established, it may well radically alter the associated clinical identity.

A textbook of medicine is thus a collection of theories about disease entities and their consequences; it is in part a nosology. If we compare Oliver Wendell Holmes's 1843 account of puerperal fever—an infection that strikes mothers after childbirth—with Thomas Sydenham's seventeenth-century description of it and with Hippocrates' description, we find a remarkable convergence. What is being described (the clinical condition of the fever) is relatively constant, but the theory behind the description has changed considerably. Theories change over time because they are produced by changes in domain assumptions, the reorganization of university curricula, professional competition among scientists, new discoveries based on laboratory trials, and technological developments.

It is not contradictory, therefore, to hold that there is a clinical reality (fever or mumps) as captured over the centuries in "classic descriptions of disease" (King 1982, 152) and that concepts of health and illness vary considerably over time, influenced by general social values, fashion, and changing social circumstances. The sociology of knowledge and the social studies of the tradition of science attempt to demonstrate that these fundamental concepts of science are socially produced. Clinical entities are also socially produced, however, by the fact, for example, that doctors are trained to recognize the signs and symptoms that, as it were, announce the presence of fever or mumps. Doctors argued for centuries about the nature and treatment of tuberculosis and constructed TB according to different paradigms, but TB continued to kill people of all social classes in large numbers (Dormandy 1999). To say that fever is socially produced is not to say that it is a fiction or that it could be conjured up by the doctor rather as a magician pulls a rabbit from a hat. The signs and symptoms of fever in a clinical setting are mediated through and by the experiences and training of physicians, however, and these physicians are the products of specific and local medical cultures. Puerperal fever killed mothers in large numbers in the first half of the nineteenth century, and it was Ignaz Semmelweis, working in Vienna General Hospital in the nineteenth century, who deduced that the infection was being transferred to mothers on the soiled hands of medical students and doctors. Doctors originally resisted Semmelweis's recommendation that they wash thoroughly in chlorinated water before inspecting mothers, because it offended their professional sense that the infections could not be caused by their behavior. The professional context and the relationship between doctors, students, and patients had an important effect on the manifestation of the problem and its resolution (R. Porter 1997, 369). Industrial and occupational injuries—such as the bone fractures, muscle strains, and the skeletal damage of professional ballet dancers—are real, but they become manifest as official injuries as a consequence of social processes and are mediated, among other things, by the norms of professional ballet (Turner and Wainwright 2003).

From a social science perspective, we can summarize the principal issues in concepts of health and illness. Regardless of the epistemological difficulties surrounding the notion of disease entities, there is widespread agreement that conceptions of disease have changed radically. Neither social scientists nor medical scientists would accept that there is a permanent and universal taxonomy of disease or that medical categories are always neutral representations of facts. The general theories of health and illness that explain the medical condition of humanity are organized according to the dominant ideologies, values, and beliefs of a culture. Medical categories are not neutral because they typically carry the metaphors of a society by which praise and blame for behavior are allocated. In addition, the nineteenth-century search for the specific etiologies of every disease, in which each disease has its own cause, has been abandoned. Theorists now see disease as having multiple, interactive causes and therefore hold that no simple, single cure is possible or desirable. The AIDS epidemic is a good illustration of this complexity. The AIDS crises in America, Russia, and Africa have very different conditions and causes, and hence there can be no single solution to the problem. In this respect, such writers as Gaston Bachelard, Kurt Goldstein, Georges Canguilhem, and Michel Foucault have influenced social science approaches that generally accept some version of the argument that sciences develop through revolutionary paradigm shifts and that scientific facts are socially constructed.

At the everyday level, social experiences of illness are equally constructed by cultural assumptions and social relationships. At this level of lay belief, there is a continuing tendency to see illness within a moral framework of blame and responsibility. This framework attempts to help individuals in a predominantly secular environment to answer questions about life and death. The growing literature, both lay and professional, on death and dying is one indication of the fact that despite or because of the erosion of the authority of traditional religious institutions, rituals, and beliefs, ordinary individuals need to find some meaning for the seemingly trivial nature of the passages from the cradle to the grave.

According to Berger's sociology of knowledge, the everyday world is constrained by certain necessary and inescapable activities: eating, sleeping, reproducing, and reciprocating. This inescapable character of the everyday world is its "facticity." These activities are clearly social, but the dull compulsion or facticity of the mundane social world is not in any meaningful or useful sense socially constructed. While breakfast as a particular time to eat is a social product, the hunger that drives us to want to eat is part of the compulsion that resides at the core of everyday routines. The ways in which we express and experience hunger are social, but suggesting that it is socially constructed does not contribute significantly to the sociological understanding of hunger. This phenomenological character of everyday life we may call the "thisness" or stuffness of existence; it is the bedrock that is resistant to social elaboration. It needs to get done. It is urgent. This world of mundane facticity, which includes the routines and events of the life process of embodiment, such as birth, maturation, and death, is a substratum that remains somewhat resistant to ideological elaboration or social construction. It is the foundation on which social construction is erected, just as labor (or practice, in the broad sense) is the base on which the superstructure is constructed. We may call this factual substratum of the everyday world the quiddity of life.

What is the relevance for health and illness of insisting on the reality of our embodiment in the everyday world? I have shown that social constructionism was an important intellectual tool of social movements, especially those movements that wanted to challenge the dominance of medical knowledge as the only possible perspective on health and illness. One issue with medical knowledge is that it applies not only to disease; a variety of other professional groups claim that medical science can also apply to a range of other human "troubles," such as misconduct. Sociologists have called the spread of medical science to human and social problems the medicalization of society. Social constructionism has been a powerful criticism of the questionable development of medical power as a foundation for knowledge of society.

My argument in this chapter has been that social constructionism has gone too far because it has virtually eliminated human embodiment by its narrow analysis of the body as a cultural object. By treating the human body as a social construct or merely a text, it has neglected the embodiment of human beings. Constructionism has examined the metaphors of the body by which medicine has organized knowledge about health and illness. The dominant metaphor of the body in the history of Western medicine has been the body as a machine (Turner 2003b). This metaphor—in which, for example, the heart is a pump—can have dangerous consequences because doctors neglect the holistic aspect of the life of the patient by treating the body as a natural object or a machine. The concept of embodiment is important because it draws attention to the integration of self and body. People do not relate to their bodies as objects because the loss of parts of the body—for example, in mastectomy—has major consequences for the sense of wholeness.

In contemporary medical science, the metaphors of the body are changing rapidly. The traditional nosological map of disease and the body is being replaced by the idea of the body as a code or as a system of information. The human genome project is an attempt to provide a comprehensive—indeed, total—map of the human genetic structure. Such new metaphors of the body will bring about fundamental changes to the ways in which disease is treated and managed, and hence they will have radical implications for the ways in which patients are perceived and treated. Advances in science do not, unfortunately, mean better management and care of patients. Better science has to be translated into better doctoring and better nursing if patients are to have better experiences of clinical and hospital care. Again, this is a further reason for emphasizing the difference between the body as a cultural construct and embodiment as an experience. The differences between the scientific view of the body and the everyday experiences of embodiment often conflict with each other. I have used an old-fashioned notion of the quiddity of illness experiences in everyday life to try to capture the separation between the mundane facts about our vulnerability as embodied people and the world of university medical science.

Chapter Three
DISEASE AND CULTURE

INTRODUCTION: THE SACRED AND PROFANE

MICHEL FOUCAULT'S *MADNESS AND CIVILIZATION* (1971) was an important contribution to the history of psychiatry because it provided a controversial challenge to the official history of the psychiatric profession. Foucault questioned the official history of the treatment of the mentally ill as a continuous evolution from a state of harmful ignorance to the benign triumph of rational science. Through an examination of the institutionalization of the insane, Foucault showed how new forms of administrative surveillance or governmentality were imposed on a heterogeneous population of the unemployed, the sick, the poor, and the socially ostracized. Psychiatric practices did not represent the liberation of the insane, but rather the institutionalization and regulation of the population to make it more productive. Medical history is often controversial because it, too, involves a hidden history of power: the struggle of more or less coherent, professional, secular, individualistic, allopathic, and predominantly private medicine to achieve dominance over a variety of rival systems. These rival and alternative systems were the religious, collective, homeopathic, alternative, complementary, and public medical systems of health care. In this brief discussion of the history of medicine, my principal concern is with both the professional exclusion of complementary and alternative medicine and the socialized public health care that depends implicitly on assumptions about social capital. To understand contemporary health care, it is important to have a historical understanding of the rise of privatized health care. Although Western, secular medicine was dominant through much of the twentieth century, health systems globally are becoming more pluralistic and fragmented. The rise of Western, scientific medicine is therefore not an evolutionary, uniform, or necessarily hegemonic development.

The professional legitimacy of scientific, allopathic, Western medicine rests in part on its epistemological claims to validity. The professional claim is that Western medicine is effective because it is based on scientific research that delivers verifiable results. In previous chapters, however, I have noted the complexity of health concepts and their contested nature. The sociology of knowledge supports the critical view that "medical facts" are clinical interpretations of medical evidence in which persuasive pronouncements require professional authority. Medical evidence is in this respect no different from sociological evidence because the data on which doctors make decisions are typically incomplete and contradictory. Facts tend to be messy and fuzzy. Health concepts are contested because, among other things, they have controversial legal, moral, and existential implications. Concepts of health and illness are closely associated with central social values because they give expression to fundamental assumptions about the ethical meaning of life and death. Descriptions of the conditions that promote health—a good diet, no tobacco use, moderate alcohol intake, physical exercise, a clean and safe environment, marriage or at least sociability, and careers that are relatively free from persistent stress—necessarily encompass "the good life" and "the good society" as well as "good health."

Because concepts of health and illness are closely associated with important social values, there are important intellectual and political battles that have surrounded the development of medical education and its institutions. Health is increasingly seen not as a collective good or as a resource but as an aspect of personal responsibility. Health education encourages an individual lifestyle in which we are encouraged to keep fit and watch our weight. The values associated with health are compatible with the general emphasis on individualism in society, but they may be less relevant to the elderly, disabled, and disadvantaged sectors of society. These individualistic values are often associated with managerial criteria that stress the importance of efficiency and cost effectiveness as the dominant criteria of medical care (Light 2001). What type of medical training and investment produces efficient, cost-effective, and beneficial outcomes? This is an important question, but we should note that two underlying assumptions result in additional questions. When we say that a health system such as the British NHS is efficient and cost effective, is this efficiency seen from the perspective of the government, the taxpayer, or the patient? When we say that medical intervention has beneficial outcomes, is that for society as a whole or from the point of view of the patient? Patients may opt for medical services that are important but expensive and inefficient from the perspective of the health service. One might argue that heart bypass surgery is desirable for elderly patients with heart conditions but may not be efficient in terms of the economic objectives of the health system as a whole. It may be that investing in an effective campaign against smoking would have more efficient and cost-effective outcomes than bypass surgery.

The use of the drug Viagra provides an instructive illustration of the controversial issues that underpin the notions of effective and beneficial medical interventions (Mamo and Fishman 2001). It also illustrates the contrast between individual needs and collective requirements. Viagra was developed unsuccessfully to treat high blood pressure, but researchers found that nitric oxide had the unintended consequence of improving erectile function. The drug was developed by Pfizer, Inc., and has been used to improve erections in men who suffer from impotence as a result, for example, of prostate cancer. There is ample evidence to suggest that sexual satisfaction is an important component of well-being among the elderly (Gott and Hinchliff 2003), and there are grounds, therefore, for medically prescribing the use of Viagra. In Britain, there have been important debates about whether Viagra should be available by prescription free of charge from the NHS.

Obviously, Viagra is a beneficial drug, but in a context of economic scarcity, should we invest in research on sexual impotence when there are many more urgent matters to resolve? Erectile dysfunction may be a source of embarrassment and disappointment, but it is not life threatening. As a drug, Viagra is beneficial to elderly men, but does it make an important medical contribution to society? In recent years, the use of Viagra has spread to many social groups and is regarded as a lifestyle drug that enhances sexual performance in men who are not otherwise experiencing dysfunction. How should we decide on the use and availability of such drugs? In some societies, medical developments are determined by a complex combination of factors: government priorities, legislation, professional goals and targets, a hierarchy of values, moral preferences, and consumer demand. In other societies, medical developments and innovations may be determined by less complex combinations: markets, profitability of companies, and consumer demand. Through the second half of the twentieth century, medical services and products were increasingly subject to market forces because there was a global trend toward the deregulation of professional and legal controls. Questions about the benefit of Viagra for individuals and its consequences for society were replaced by a more basic question: who will pay for it?

Conceptions of health originally arose out of fundamental religious and moral views about existence, and differences in orientation toward health reflect basic structural and cultural differences in power relations in society. In traditional societies, the contrast between health and illness was a fundamental principle of social classification and was closely connected to the distinction between the sacred and the profane (Durkheim 1954). Beliefs about health and illness were inextricably bound up with religious notions of the sacredness of the body in terms of purity and danger. Primitive notions of pollution and taboo were not related to hygiene because there was simply no secular knowledge of principles of cleanliness (M. Douglas 1966). For example, the dietary prescriptions of the Hebrew Bible relating to pork are recommendations about appropriate religious, not hygienic, behavior. In the classificatory system of the Hebrew Bible, animals that ruminate, such as cows, typically have cloven feet. Pigs have cloven feet, however, but they do not ruminate and so they are difficult to classify. They are forbidden and used to conceptualize anomalies in social life. Anthropologists have shown us how pigs raise fundamental questions in the Hebrew Bible's theology about the nature of the universe. Such concepts about purity were directed at the "health" of social relationships, within which the individual, not the body, was located.

A taboo, which divides the world into the acceptable and the unacceptable through the contrast between the edible and the inedible, is a conceptual mechanism for giving the world structure and meaning. People became sick not because of a breach of hygienic regulations but because they had transgressed a social norm, or taboo, that separated the sacred from the profane. Sickness and health were often associated with taboos on bodily fluids, where contact—for example, with menstrual blood—could cause illness in an individual or disaster for the tribe. The Inuit explained personal misfortune, illness, and failure to catch food in terms of transgressions of taboos, typically those surrounding the ritualistic organization of menstruation (Turner 2003b). Both these misfortunes and these sicknesses were treated through shamanistic practices such as seances, at which a "confession" took place to purify the individual and the group.

In such a system of meaning, sickness was associated with evil forces that attack human beings through, for instance, witchcraft and demonic possession. Concepts of illness functioned within a cosmology of good and evil, and they were explanatory devices that described and possibly justified evil and misery. Notions of illness have typically been set within a general theodicy, a system of beliefs that attempts to explain and justify the presence of human disease and suffering. When people fall victim of disease and sickness, there is almost inevitably the question, why me? Concepts of health and disease have typically provided an answer to questions of misfortune, and thus the dominant assumptions of disease have been located within a discourse of sacred phenomena.

With the process of modernization, concepts of health and illness are transferred to more secular paradigms and are eventually embraced by various scientific discourses. Health and illness have moved within the classificatory paradigm of society. In Western medicine, disease entities become increasingly differentiated, and disease states become more specific as the human body is itself differentiated into its component parts. The human genome project offers new classificatory opportunities. Microbiology provides an account of viruses, which invade the body and have no explicit connection with the moral or religious status of the individual.

As scientific concepts of disease replaced traditional notions of the religious character of illness, the social status of the medical professional increased, and the status and role of traditional healers—medicine men, wise women, and midwives—declined. In addition, a differentiation developed between physical and mental health that in turn relied on a basic division between mind and body. This mind-body dualism was associated with the empiricist revolution in philosophy that came to be called rationalist Cartesianism. The idea that there is a profound division between mind and body was associated with the seventeenth-century rationalist philosophy of René Descartes, from whom modern science derived the basic ideas of Cartesianism. The idea of "mental illness" was subsequently elaborated by separate developments in clinical psychology, psychiatry, and psychoanalysis (Busfield 2000). Finally, the social sciences of health and illness are themselves part of the growing complexity of the contemporary model of sickness, in which medical sociology and public health address the social dimensions of sickness through the concept of the sick role (Turner 1995a, 5).

The historical development of concepts of health and illness in Western societies is characterized by increasing secularization, the rise of scientific theories of health, the separation of mental and physical illness, the erosion of traditional therapies by scientific practices, and the differentiation of categories into specific micro notions. Secular Western medicine spread through Africa and Asia, especially where Britain established Commonwealth teaching hospitals. There was a cultural process involving the colonization of indigenous belief systems by Western, professional medicine (Arnold 2000).

The official history of medicine is thus a progressive and inevitable development in which empirically valid knowledge has replaced invalid, bogus medical ideas. Historical accounts of medicine are typically triumphal narratives of the progressive employment of technology and scientific knowledge to replace traditional systems whose therapeutic achievements were at best merely placebo effects. Even a critical history of the medical profession such as Roy Porter's *Bodies Politic* (2001) treated the rise of British medicine as a triumph over quacks, bonesetters, naturalists, homeopaths, and wise women. These accounts often fail to register the continuous struggle among competing medical systems for social dominance and fail to notice the growing pluralism and complexity of the modern system of medicine and health care. There are various reasons for doubting the final hegemonic triumph of allopathic medicine over its historical rivals.

Although there has been a general trend toward secularized medicine, it is important not to exaggerate the homogeneity of traditional medical systems. There existed, even in premodern medical systems, considerable complexity and dispute. For example, there were radical differences between Plato, Aristotle, Erasistratus, and Galen as to the nature of the human body, its functions and structure, and the purpose of medicine (Cunningham 1997). There is also no neat point in history when secular views became dominant. While the sixteenth-century anatomical works of Andreas Vesalius were seen to pave the way toward scientific medicine, Vesalius clearly retained the religious view that the ultimate role of medicine is to reveal the hand of God in nature. Such medical sciences remained an important part of natural philosophy, the branch of knowledge that exhibits the laws of God. As such, scientific medicine frequently carried an overt moral and religious message.

The lay public has not passively accepted the authority of secular and scientifically trained doctors, and complementary and alternative medical systems have always thrived alongside Western allopathic medicine. In the twentieth century, there was a great revival of alternative systems of medicine and widespread criticism of the claims of allopathic medicine. There are considerable philosophical and ethical problems with the role of hegemonic, scientific medicine, which cannot be regarded as a single, unified, and complete account of disease. We should not accept an official version of medical history as the heroic march of reason through history, resulting in the final triumph of rational science over magical or irrational systems of medicine (Vaughan 1991). For example, the Mexican health system, created in 1943, gave a central role to biomedical, allopathic, secular medicine. Although law permitted homeopathy and chiropractic, they were never practiced in public hospitals. While there has been an official system with the support of the state, alternative nonbiomedical systems have flourished (Nigenda et al. 2001). Pluralism has grown because alternative medical provision—faith healing, homeopathy, traditional medicine, herbalism, and so forth—is seen to be cheaper, to have fewer negative side effects, to be less intrusive, and to establish better psychological rapport with the patient. Pluralism is of course not confined to Mexico; it is a consequence of consumer demand for different medical services and global economic pressures for the deregulation of all services.

The development of medicine is often understood in terms of a "divided legacy" (Coulter 1977), namely, a struggle between intervening in nature to change the pattern of disease and working with nature to bring about healing. The former method is associated with allopathic medicine and the latter with homeopathy. The history of homeopathy is particularly important for comprehending the struggle to establish political dominance over the market of professional health care and cure. In the early nineteenth century, Samuel Hahnemann developed homeopathy not as an attack on the rise of scientific medicine but rather as an alternative to aggressive and often brutal forms of medical intervention (May and Sirur 1998). As a therapeutic, its aim was always to replace polypharmacy—the use of multiple drugs—with single, diluted drugs to concentrate on the patient's unique manifestation of symptoms and to extinguish the natural disease with an "artificial disease." The principle of homeopathy is curing like with like (*similia simi-libus curentur*). Because the dilution of drugs requires testing the effects of homeopathy at a submolecular level, homeopathy presents peculiar problems in terms of the normal processes of medical evaluation. Despite considerable scientific criticism, homeopathy in Britain was never successfully subordinated to allopathic medicine, where it has enjoyed the support of members of the royal family. Homeopathic hospitals in Liverpool, London, Glasgow, and Bristol were eventually incorporated into the NHS. Since the 1980s, there has been growing interest in homeopathic treatment among junior doctors. Because training programs for general practice have increasingly emphasized the importance of communication skills, homeopathy, which has traditionally noted the importance of listening to the personal experience of illness, is highly compatible with the professional norms of personal care.

Complementary and alternative medicine has grown in popularity, but it is often either co-opted by or subordinated to allopathic biomedical systems. The public health movement represents an important and persistent challenge to the apparent dominance of individualistic, allopathic, secular medicine, however, partly because it appeals to the same paradigm of scientific evidence to substantiate its claims. The claims of public health research and its advocacy of preventive medicine are supported by social epidemiology, demography, and the social sciences. The growth of collectivist and secular assumptions about health and illness was characteristic of the public health movements of the nineteenth century, when radicals like Friedrich Engels, Edwin Chadwick, and Rudolf Virchow identified the causes of human disease in the deprivations and alienation of working-class slums in a rapidly expanding urban environment. In this study of medical sociology, I have identified Virchow as a radical social critic whose medical reports paved the way for the political economy of health and the importance of social capital as a general model of health and illness, but he was also the founder of cell research as a scientific basis for pathology (Taylor and Rieger 1984). His 1858 *Cellular Pathology* was a major development in medicine and resulted in the reform of departments of pathology around Europe (Clendening 1942). Advocates of public health reform are not necessarily critical of laboratory-based science or evidence-based medicine, but they assume that investment in such public utilities as clean water and adequate housing is more efficient and effective than investment in training doctors to provide individualized, allopathic medicine in a profit-driven health market. Public health reformers recognize the need for doctors, but they put the emphasis of health policy on improvements in the social environment.

Nineteenth-century social reformers described disease as a collective and secular condition of social existence in emergent capitalism, where morbidity and mortality rates were directly related to the quality of the social environment—housing, food and water, sanitation, and income levels. In the twentieth century, similar concepts of health and illness were embraced by radical medical sociologists like Howard Waitzkin (1983) and Vicente Navarro (1976) and by radical historians of medicine like Henry E. Sigerist (1951) and his students (Fee and Brown 1997). These approaches to disease are very different from the individualist, secular concepts that form the basis of allopathic medicine and empiricist Cartesian science. Allopathic medical traditions legitimate significant medical interventions in the life of individuals. Sickness is treated as an effect of disease entities such as bacteria or viruses or as an organic pathology. Health improves with isolation from germs and viruses, with personal hygiene, and with medical intervention by surgery, by professional doctors and their research universities, and by medical faculties and general hospitals.

In contemporary medicine, genetic explanations of health and illness are transforming existing causal paradigms (Smart 2003). With individualized medicine, private health insurance is a crucial responsibility of the patient if he or she wants an effective response to acute conditions. By contrast, socialized medicine has been opposed by critics who argue that public provision reduces individual responsibility and increases the burden of the "undeserving poor" on the taxpayer and the state. The arguments in favor of preventive and public health interventions have been based on the historical epidemiology and political economy of such works as Thomas McKeown's *Role of Medicine* (1979), Richard Wilkinson's *Unhealthy Societies* (1996), and Vicente Navarro's *Crisis, Health, and Medicine* (1986), which broadly established the argument that social factors such as housing, income, and education determine health and illness and that medical interventions such as vaccination begin to have an effect only after a society has achieved a relatively high level of general wealth. Neoconservative critics of the argument will claim that in societies that have already achieved high standards of wealth, such as the United States, the health needs of the population are best served by a system that combines individualized, scientific medical services, consumer choice, medical pluralism, and private insurance. In order to understand these conflicts, we need to understand how modern medicine evolved historically.

DESCARTES AND MEDICAL SCIENCE

In the seventeenth century, there emerged an "elective affinity" between the ascetic and individualistic ethic of the Protestant sects and the emergent culture of competitive capitalism (Weber 1930). Alongside the growth of rational capitalism, there emerged an elective affinity between the seventeenth-century philosophies of René Descartes and Isaac Newton, and empirical and rational medicine. The development of experimental medicine was founded on their rationalism through the work of the eighteenth-century physician Hermann Boerhaave. Just as early capitalism assumed an individualistic and ascetic orientation, so the medical revolution of the seventeenth and early eighteenth centuries acquired an individualistic, rational, and experimental ethos. There was an important convergence in values and practice in the Protestant Reformation, Cartesian science, and medicine.

Descartes created the basis of modern experimental rationalism by attempting, through a thought experiment, to exclude religious and irrational dimensions from philosophy. Descartes's rationalist philosophy was the foundation of Cartesianism, which separates mind and body, and promoted the experimental method. His rationalism attempted to find a point of certainty that was beyond further doubt. His philosophical system rested on the famous individualist slogan *cogito ergo sum,* "I am thinking, therefore I exist." The force of this claim is to give a primacy to cognitive rationalism over the senses, and it established the priority of mind over matter. Descartes was not entirely successful in establishing his own brand of rationalist philosophy in the universities, which was being replaced by an empirical philosophy that was mechanical and Newtonian. By the end of the seventeenth century, rationalist medicine was neo-Newtonian. Cartesian rationalism as a system remained a profoundly influential doctrine, however. Cartesian secularism became a potent aspect of medical belief. It required a simple and complete separation between mind and body. Indeed, in Cartesianism, body is merely an extension of mind.

Cartesian rationalism was combined with Newtonian physics in the quest for a mathematical system to express the laws that govern the human body. Physicians sought to create a medical system that would have the same elegance and simplicity as the Newtonian laws of gravity. Physicians like Archibald Pitcairne in the early eighteenth century were part of a scientific network stretching from Edinburgh, in Scotland, through Oxford to Leiden, in the Netherlands, a scientific network that wanted to provide medical theory with mathematical certainty (Guerrini 1989). This theory was referred to as *principiia medicinae theoreticae mathematicae*. The physicians' influence was considerable. Newtonian ideas became important in the work of George Cheyne, whose early-eighteenth-century publications on diet had a considerable impact among the London elite (Turner 1982). Cheyne offered medical advice to the London coffeehouse set, who, like Cheyne, were victims of obesity. The principal causes of melancholy were connected to excessive consumption of food, drink, and tobacco and to a sedentary lifestyle. While Cheyne was a practical man and wanted to use diet as a method of improving the mental state of his patients, he was also Newtonian in understanding the body as a system of pumps whose flows could be understood with mathematical certainty. His status as a doctor was greatly enhanced by his scientific vision of the body as a hydraulic system.

Philosophers of the period reduced God to a clockmaker who is in a general way responsible for the functioning of the Newtonian universe but does not intervene directly in the lives of human beings. The iatromathematicians wanted to analyze the human body with the same precision that Newton had achieved in the natural environment. William Harvey had discovered the principles of the circulation of blood, validating the doctrine of circulation on Aristotelian and teleological grounds. His 1649 *Anatomical Exercise on the Circulation of the Blood* gave further authority to the view of the human body as a mechanical pump whose flows and tides could be measured mathematically by exact calculation. The machine might need a soul to start the motor, but there was little room for a reflexive mind in this mechanical universe.

We should not exaggerate the secular dimension of medical practice in the seventeenth century. Medical interventions were still typically set within a broader moral and religious framework. In prescribing a dietary regime in order to control the machine, Cheyne was following a long line of Christian physicians who sought to regulate the soul through a diet of the body. His views on living a disciplined life to control the nerves appealed to the leader of Methodism, John Wesley, who in his 1747 *Primitive Physick* provided a Methodist version of the medical regime. In addition, the moral and religious significance of the seventeenth-century anatomy lesson should not be underestimated. Comparative anatomy had always raised questions of conscience, because it was thought to spy on God's secret construction of the universe or to be a vain and pointless quest for ultimate causes. From a Christian point of view, if the body is merely flesh, can the anatomical inquiry reveal anything of God's purpose? Anatomy had, as a result, remained a conservative area of medical science, where it continued to be dominated by Galen's *On the Conduct of Anatomy*. Anatomy had begun to change radically with the work of Andreas Vesalius, who, through experimentation on human beings, broke away from the scholastic conformity to the Galenic tradition. Whereas the authority of Galenic medicine rested on the ancient traditions of academic scholarship within the universities, the experimental attitude of Vesalius was radical because it was based on direct observations.

In the seventeenth century, the anatomy lesson continued to function as a moral lesson. In the work of anatomists like the sixteenth-century Andreas Laurentius, the observer was encouraged to "know thyself" and to embrace the feeling that "there but for the grace of God, go I." These sentiments are well illustrated in Rembrandt's famous 1632 painting of *The Anatomy Lesson of Dr. Nicolaas Tulp,* which shows Tulp in the Waaggebouw in Amsterdam with the sectioned body of the criminal Aris Kint. The picture has many iconic features pointing to Christian truths about the frailty and finitude of human beings. For example, behind the figure of Tulp, in the wall, is a shell, a Christian symbol of baptism. The anatomy lesson continued to be part of a moral discourse about sinfulness and judgment within the new framework of scientific experimentation that stood at the core of the seventeenth-century scientific revolution.

Foucault and Panoptic Surveillance

Contemporary sociological analysis of medical systems has been profoundly influenced by the work of Foucault. His research on systems of knowledge follows the tradition of such philosophers of science as Gaston Bachelard and Georges Canguilhem, who demonstrated that scientific revolutions often take the form of a violent break with the past—an "epistemological rupture"—and that science is best understood in its practice rather than in its claims, which are typically inconsistent with, or not supported by, its practical applications. Both propositions tend to be critical of perspectives that treat history as a smooth and continuous progress. Cartesianism is a scientific rupture that was important in the development of Foucault's historical understanding of mental health. Descartes had ruled out the possibility that madness could invalidate the claim "I am thinking, therefore I exist." His exclusion of insanity matched the exclusion of the insane from normal society. The fantastic ship of fools was imagined in creative literature as a vessel to carry the insane away from society, in the belief that the rocking of the waves would calm their troubled minds, but ships were actually used to exclude the insane from society. In Frankfurt in 1399, seamen were instructed by the townsfolk to remove a naked lunatic from the city. The philosophical exclusion of madness paralleled the social seclusion of the insane.

Foucault (1971) identified an administrative transformation in the mid seventeenth century when large numbers of people were confined in detention in such places as the General Hospital in Paris. Because the definition of madness was broad and vague, detention functioned as a way of regulating the poor, needy, and incompetent. "Madness" was a regulatory discourse for the management of large populations. A second break occurred in the eighteenth century when "madness" as an indefinite concept began to give way to modern notions of "mental illness." Whereas madness, which was equivalent to folly or foolishness in Shakespeare's *King Lear,* was historically associated with divine insight and creativity, mental illness became a technical discourse, which was overtly separated from more traditional notions of possession, violence, and creativity. In the folly of King Lear, reason and madness could communicate, but the modern notion of insanity has domesticated and neutralized the old forces of jest and foolishness. This new conception of mental illness required a different setting, and Foucault traced the evolution of psychiatry alongside the institutional growth of the modern asylum, which applied the principles of panoptic surveillance from the utilitarianism of Bentham to the management of the mentally ill (1977).

Foucault's history of the categories of mental health criticized the dominant ideology of psychiatry, which interpreted the history of its own profession as the triumph of reason over witchcraft and magic. Foucault noted that like medieval responses to witchcraft, psychiatry involved various forms of governmentality to regulate individuals whose behavior was in various ways regarded as deviant. His approach directed attention to the function of concepts of disease and illness as components of a larger system of social regulation. Although his approach was very different in its assumptions and methods, there is some similarity between Foucault and Thomas Szasz (1961, 1970), who claimed that the practice of psychiatry eroded individual and human rights. According to Szasz, the differences between liberal democracy and Communist authoritarianism had been exaggerated, because in both societies such medical practices as electroconvulsive therapy could be used to control political dissidents. The importance of writers like Foucault and Szasz in the social science of medicine was to raise fundamental questions about the alleged neutrality and reliability of scientific method and concepts in the management of human affairs, because the medicalization of deviance often removed the right of an individual to rational debate. The attempt to treat homosexuality as a mental disease is the classic illustration.

GERM THEORY AND INFECTIOUS DISEASES

Although the nineteenth century is seen in official histories of medicine as the great triumph of the scientific revolution, it also disguised a profound struggle between professional allopathic medicine and the social medicine of the public health movement (Turner 2000a). At the core of this debate was, on the one hand, the great success of scientific responses to infection by means of such techniques as vaccination and, on the other hand, the chronic social needs of the urban poor and the response of social science in the form of town planning. This division is a classic illustration of the historical conflict between the view that environmental pollution and social degradation determine morbidity and mortality and the emphasis on doctors' treating individual patients with medical interventions grounded in scientific discovery. These differences are particularly important in the historical analysis of such epidemics as tuberculosis (Szreter 1988). Were the major improvements in health a consequence of medical intervention to control disease by means of vaccination, or were the improvements in health a function of rising standards of living? The nineteenth century produced monumental social investigations of the conditions of the poor that continue to influence social responses to health and illness.

Throughout Europe, there were major social attempts to control illness through the political manipulation of urban conditions to improve hygiene. For example, in the Netherlands from 1840 to 1890, the Hygienists—a group of medical practitioners—embraced the view that the health of the nation was determined by public health. The Hygienists rejected attempts to centralize public health at the level of the state and supported some devolution of health care. The movement illustrates the fact that medical and political reform tend to go together, because the Hygienists were very much a product of the 1848 liberal revolutions characteristic of Germany and France. In their medical views, they rejected assumptions about contagion and the traditional methods of describing diseases by their external aspects, which were typical of early nineteenth-century epidemiology. These concepts were focused on ontology. For the Hygienists, diseases are not entities that flourish and die, following environmental changes, but are caused by anatomical and physiological relations in the body. By their standardization of disease classification, they were able to collect effective statistical evidence on morbidity and mortality. After 1850, they came to accept the *Bodentheorie* (ground, or soil, theory) of Max von Pettenkofer, a professor of hygiene who claimed that epidemics were caused by soil pollution. His reputation was based on his analysis of the South German cholera epidemic of 1854. The cholera germ was a product of the soil, not the human intestine; Pettenkofer offered a technical solution, a reconstruction of urban water systems in order to regulate water levels. The *Bodentheorie* was well suited to the political culture of postrevolutionary Europe because it implied a technical rather than a political response to epidemics.

This illustration of public health in the nineteenth-century Netherlands belongs within the broader context of the debate about contagion. The notion that disease was passed from one person to another by infective organisms—that is, by contagion—can be traced to responses to pestilence in early societies. The author of Leviticus recognized that leprosy and gonorrhea were transmitted by contagion and therefore had to be quarantined—a name derived from *quarantena,* or the forty-day period of isolation required of people entering Italian ports who were thought to be infected by disease. The alternative view of epidemics was that they are caused by atmospheric influence, or "epidemic miasma." Epidemics are caused by bad air (*mala aria*). Although the notion of miasma was long ago discredited by the discovery of the living organisms that produce many diseases, it recognized poor living conditions and lack of hygiene as causes of illness. The theory of contagion by infective organisms also led, after much professional resistance, to the conclusion that disease is spread by doctors from one patient to another. Semmelweis's 1860s puerperal fever work was significant in the development of hygienic practices in the treatment of mothers. Also in the nineteenth century, Joseph Lister, building on the tradition of Louis Pasteur and Robert Koch, eventually supplied the scientific principles behind these practical procedures. These advances made possible a much safer environment for the practice of surgery and contributed to the containment of infections following hospitalization. Despite the medical profession's resistance to the scientific discoveries of Semmelweis and Lister, the advances in medical science made possible the growth of medicine as a "learned profession" driven by the cutting edge of science.

THE FLEXNER REPORT AND THE MEDICINAL CURRICULUM

The twentieth century was the context for radical changes in medicine. In those changes, one cannot separate transformations of the concepts of health and illness from the development of the role of professional medicine (Stevens 1998). Doctoring before the rise of medical science, the medical school, and professional closure had more to do with social drama than with science (R. Porter 2001). The everyday world of the eighteenth century was shaped by the constant risk of injury and disease, to which women and children were especially vulnerable. Mothers and infants suffered from puerperal and dysenteric fevers, and two-fifths of children perished before they reached five years of age. Gout, rheumatism, and respiratory complaints were the common companions of the elderly, and with the development of industrial capitalism, so-called filth diseases and tuberculosis became the persistent scourges of rich and poor alike. Medical practice had little to offer in terms of effective and reliable therapies or cures. Traditional medicine did not have what we would regard as specific, determinate medical outcomes. Rather, it offered a medical rhetoric that gave the uncertainties of life a meaning and developed a public drama of disaster, disease, and death. Medicine was constituted by a set of cultural practices that can be understood within a ritualistic, spiritual, and aesthetic framework. Medical interventions had consequences insofar as they had placebo effects. The placebo effect, an important component of the therapeutic process, depended on the doctor's theatrical performance and the imaginative receptivity of the patient. Doctors and preachers were part of a common ritualistic system that offered meaning and compensation.

If there was a distinctive and well-defined doctor's role, there was a corresponding patient's role. In the absence of a scientific and tested paradigm of scientific medicine, doctor and patient shared a language and a body of knowledge. Before the development of pathological anatomy, diagnostic technologies, and germ theory, it was typically the patient, not the doctor, who spelled out the nature of the complaint and its possible solutions. The theatrical features of the clinical encounter were stage-managed by the patient, and hence the patient's condition had to be negotiated. The sick role can often give great psychological comfort to a patient by making him or her the center of attention within the family, and invalidism and hypochondria became popular topics of the eighteenth-century novel. Excessive bile and hypochondria were common conditions of people with talent and imagination. In Britain, inland health spas at Bath, Buxton, and Cheltenham and seaside resorts at Brighton and Scarborough flourished as recreation centers for the rich and their physicians. The image of the early-Victorian doctor as the debonair gentleman evolved to meet the new heath craze of bathing in, and occasionally drinking, seawater. Before the professional development of the medical school, medicine was a liberal profession, surgery was merely a manual art, and pharmacists were merely shopkeepers. Rivalry and acrimonious conflicts within the professional body served only to inflate lay distrust.

The Victorian period was one of steady reform, however. In Britain, the reconstruction of the medical profession was not fully achieved until the Medical Act of 1858, which established a single Medical Register under the auspices of a General Medical Council, thereby consolidating the status of doctors vis-à-vis their rivals. While the act created an organized profession, general practitioners remained underpaid and overworked. They were forced to be civil to their socially superior patients and to tolerate slow payments and bad debts. The doctor became an idealized figure—educated, long-suffering, poor, compassionate, and the servant of his community.

The transformation of the university curriculum indicated shifting balances in authority between different professional groups and institutions. The reform of the medical curriculum is an important guide to these changes. The triumph of allopathic, individualist, and secular medicine over social or environmental medicine was symbolized by the publication of the Flexner Report—*Medical Education in the United States and Canada*—in 1910. Abraham Flexner, a secondary-school educator with no medical education, prepared for his inquiry by meeting the faculty of the John Hopkins University School of Medicine (Rothstein 1987, 144). Flexner argued that scientific medicine requires intensive and protracted university-based training in the fundamental natural science curriculum. The immediate implication was that only students from the upper classes could achieve the lengthy university training necessary for entry into professional medical roles (Berliner 1984). The report had the consequence of limiting the flow of black students, women, and the working class into the medical faculty, and the recruitment of these groups into the profession showed no sign of revival in North America until after 1970 (Mumford 1983).

The Flexner Report recognized and authorized the social dominance of a research-oriented scientific medicine, in which the biological sciences, along with laboratory training, provide the foundation of medical understanding. Allopathic medicine triumphed over complementary medicine generally and homeopathic medicine in particular (Rothstein 1987). Medicine was increasingly specialized, and a division of labor emerged to deal with the separate organs of the body. This new breed of scientific doctors consisted of specialists in the biological functioning of the human body.

Simultaneously, the medical faculty in the university system evolved as a separate, high-cost research faculty with its own authority and eventual dominance over the academic board. Medical faculties were increasingly separate, in spatial and academic terms, from the rest of the university. This phenomenon reinforced the social solidarity of the medical faculty and effectively isolated the medical curriculum from other parts of the university. Specialization and subspecialization intensified the technical aspects of the scientific discourse of medicine that was later associated with the rapid growth of physiology and pharmacology. These curriculum changes laid the foundation for the golden age of twentieth-century scientific medicine and the domination of the Flexner reforms, which lasted until the 1970s.

The growing importance of the general hospital was also associated with the rising social status of medicine. Improvements in hygiene, sanitation, and nursing resulted in declining morbidity rates, making hospitals safe for their middle-class clients. The growth of scientific medicine, the advent of the research medical faculty, and the evolution of the hospital created a distinctive period of medical professionalization in which the medical associations controlled entry into the medical occupational cluster (Larson 1977). Complementary processes of professionalization occurred in dentistry, pharmacy, nursing, and many other paraprofessional groupings. These social changes ushered in the era of the medical-industrial complex (Ehrenreich and Ehrenreich 1970) and fostered a new wave of social criticism directed at the negative consequences of the "medicalization of society" and the growth of iatrogenic illness, or illness that is an unintended consequence of medical intervention (Illich 1977).

A variety of medical analysts have argued that since the 1970s there has been a profound transformation of health-care systems, which has been associated with a decline in the centrality of professional medicine and its professional autonomy (Starr 1982). The decline of medical dominance has also been associated with the erosion of social security plans, centralized welfare states, and the commercialization of medical provision. As insurance companies have come to influence debates about and policies on health funding, the professional autonomy of doctors has been constrained. Governments have also turned to a mixture of preventive medicine, third-sector finance, and public health policies to support self-regulation. The fiscal crises in health care are closely related to the graying of the population, because people over sixty-five years of age suffer from higher rates of morbidity and hence place a greater burden on health-care services. This economic burden is also associated with the fact that in modern societies more old people live alone and therefore cannot call on relatives for support. These political and economic changes have focused the attention of medical sociologists on governmentality (Turner 1997c).

THE MCKEOWN THESIS AND SOCIAL MEDICINE

By the second half of the twentieth century, there was general agreement that the great epoch of infectious disease had come to an end. Medical historians and epidemiologists like Thomas McKeown (1979) looked back on the nineteenth century and argued that the infectious scourges of the previous century (TB, measles, whooping cough, and venereal disease) had virtually disappeared as improvements were made in housing, water supply, food, and education. His thesis, which is not confined to the nineteenth century, demonstrates the importance of environmental and social causes in the decline of mortality rates. TB was declining steadily from the 1830s, before the use of bacillus Calmette-Guerin vaccination and the introduction of drug treatment such as streptomycin in 1944, para-aminosalicylic acid in 1946, and isoniazid in 1952. The drug treatment of TB had a profound impact on mortality rates. Whereas nine hundred girls died from TB in England and Wales in 1946, only nine died in 1961. According to McKeown, however, these improvements were consequences of socioeconomic changes, which enhanced the general health status of the population.

Social inequality and poverty are now regarded as major determinants of individual health and of major differences in morbidity and mortality between social classes, as demonstrated, for example, in Great Britain's Black Report (Townsend and Davidson 1982). With the creation of the welfare state in Britain after the Second World War, it was assumed that British society was becoming more egalitarian, but in 1980 the Black Report, on class differences in health, showed large differences between occupational classes. Standardized death rates for social classes I (professional groups) and V (unskilled manual occupations) indicated that a salaried professional person would live just over seven years longer than a working-class person (Wilkinson 1986, 1). These investigations into class and health gave social medicine a critical vision of society. In 1944, the Goodenough Committee (the Interdepartmental Committee on Medical Schools) asserted that social medicine involves disease prevention rather than simply treatment; it regarded health promotion rather than therapy as the primary duty of a doctor; it emphasized the "social environment"; and it recognized that personal problems of health could have communal as well as individual dimensions (D. Porter 1997). In Britain, the new discipline of social medicine was advanced by radicals like John Ryle, who in 1942 became the first professor of social medicine. Social medicine, as a result, has often been closely connected with political radicalism, because it has concluded that poverty causes illness and therefore the remedy has to be sought in social change, even radical political change. By contrast, general medicine was focused on curing diseases and treating individuals rather than looking at the social causes that promote health. In North America, the debate about the social causes of illness and disease was promoted by medical sociologists like Howard Waitzkin, who explored the notion of "the second sickness," a disease of the body produced by social injustice (Waitzkin 1983; Waitzkin and Waterman 1974).

As mortality rates fell, the populations of the industrial societies increased while birth rates remained high. Demographic transition resulted, however, as contraceptive devices became more common and a new emphasis fell on the family and motherhood. People sought to control their reproduction, and birth rates began to decline. The conventional view is that modernization, in demographic terms, involves an S-shaped curve as societies pass from high death and birth rates to low death and birth rates. One further consequence, in the absence of migration, is the graying of the population as deaths from infectious diseases are replaced by mortality from cancer, heart disease, and strokes. As Western societies became more affluent, geriatric illnesses, such as diabetes, began to dominate the demography. In terms of social knowledge, social gerontology developed and remains an incoherent domain of theory relating to both individual and cohort aging (B. S. Green 1993). The aging of the population has also given rise to a general debate about the impact of age dependency on the capacity of societies to provide care in old age. The new social gerontology has begun to chronicle a wide range of new infirmities and misfortunes awaiting people who have successfully survived into later life—for example, Alzheimer's disease, which is present in 20 percent of the population over age eighty-five.

Although geriatric treatment has not enjoyed the same status as heroic medical intervention in acute diseases, there has been considerable interest in a range of degenerative conditions. For example, there has been a medicalization of "women's complaints," especially menopause (Barker 1998). There has been considerable debate about the existence and consequences of premenstrual syndrome, the universality of menopause, and the sexual drive in old age. Some anthropologists have denied that menopause is universal, claiming that maturation for women in many societies, including Japan, is not accompanied by hot flashes, tension, and irritability (Lock 1993). Medical responses, such as HRT, have been equally controversial, with accusations that similar aging processes in men have been ignored or neglected. There has been a political backlash to what is perceived as an imbalance in investment in research into men's health. Many activist men's groups argue that given the political importance of feminism, men's diseases—such as prostate cancer, which is the second leading cause of death from cancer in older men in the United States—have been neglected.

The graying of the population of the United States, where in 1990 more than 12 percent of the population was over sixty-five, has resulted in important political conflicts over illness categories. With medicalization, there is a tendency to treat aging as a disease rather than an inevitable and natural process. With profound medical interventions—cosmetic surgery, HRT, organ transplants, and heart bypass surgery—aging can be partially arrested. While the rich and the famous have attempted to deny aging and death, mainstream gray politics has challenged the assumption that immobility, memory loss, and an erosion of libidinal interest are inevitable consequences of aging (Friedan 1993).

THE CONSEQUENCES OF GLOBALIZATION: THE NEW PLAGUES

By the 1970s, it was assumed that the conquest of disease in Western societies would require the development of drugs that would delay or manage old age. As medical attention moved from acute to chronic diseases, preventive medicine and health education focused on the containment of diabetes and heart disease. This complacency was shattered in the 1980s by the emergence of the epidemic of HIV/AIDS, which was first reported in 1979 and 1980. HIV spread rapidly among the homosexual communities of North America, Europe, and Australia. The epidemic has, and will have, a major economic impact on third world societies and on those societies—such as Islamic fundamentalist societies—that refuse to recognize the presence of HIV-positive people in their midst. HIV is now reported in 130 countries, and millions of people carry the virus. In North America, HIV and AIDS were originally confined to the homosexual communities of the West Coast and New York City. In Australia, approximately 80 percent of new cases are reported in Sydney, the gay capital of the continent. HIV subsequently spread to heterosexual couples, however, and to drug users who share needles. The epidemic often gave rise to hostile moral condemnation of gay men, demonstrating once more the intimate connection between medical and moral discourses.

I refer to the HIV/AIDS phenomenon as an epidemic partly to indicate its complexity. One does not die of AIDS but from a cluster of resulting conditions, such as pneumonia. AIDS is a medical condition that produces a spectrum of illnesses and discomforts, and so understanding AIDS requires recognition of other "opportunistic infections." The constellation of signs and symptoms in the context of HIV infection is termed the AIDS-related complex, or ARC. In short, AIDS is socially constructed out of the multiplicity of illnesses and malignancies that opportunistically flourish on a depleted immune system. Given the complexity of the condition, it is not surprising that a wealth of social metaphors also multiplied. Susan Sontag (1989) lists a few of these metaphors, among them an invasion like medieval plagues and pollution resulting from personal perversity.

Sexually transmitted diseases have forced society to rethink policies on infectious disease, but they have also demonstrated once more that medical understanding can never easily be separated from moral assumptions about "normal" behavior. AIDS has also indicated that the development of human health will be inevitably and inextricably part of a more general process of cultural globalization. In previous centuries, plagues were spread by migration and trade, but diseases generally remained specific to geographic niches. With the growth of world tourism and trade, the global risk of infectious disease has increased rapidly. Influenza epidemics now spread almost instantaneously. There is widespread anxiety about the development of a variety of new conditions that are difficult to diagnose and classify, complex in their function and diffusion, and resistant to rapid or conventional treatments. The list of such conditions includes the eruption of newly discovered diseases, such as hantavirus; the migration of diseases to new areas, such as cholera in Latin America; diseases produced by new technologies, such as toxic shock syndrome and Legionnaires' disease; and diseases that spread from animals to humans, such as SARS. The West Nile virus (WNV) arrived in New York in 1999, and the epidemic is growing as it moves westward. WNV is expected in densely populated areas of California in 2004, where mosquitoes are efficient carriers of the virus. In 20 percent of cases, victims develop fevers, and in the elderly the brain can become infected. In 2002, the virus caused 4,156 confirmed cases and 284 deaths. These problems have, along with Ebola, Marburg virus, Lassa fever, and swine flu, generated a concern for "the coming plague" (I. Garrett 1995).

These fears have been associated with the perception that we now face a new generation of hazards and risks that arise from the global pollution of the atmosphere and the environment. Global hazards gave rise to a new theory of society in the work of Ulrich Beck (1992), who argued that we have moved, along with modernization, into an uncertain and precarious social condition, which he called "risk society." As society becomes more sophisticated, the potential risks from scientific experimentation increase, especially where medical innovations are inadequately regulated. Indeed, as societies become increasingly deregulated and subject only to market discipline, the scale of the risks and hazards increases. Many critical commentators claim that the damage from the thalidomide drug, the spread of bovine spongiform encephalopathy (BSE, or "mad cow disease"), and the speculation surrounding the causes of variant Creutzfeldt-Jakob disease (vCJD) are evidence of the arrival of a risk society in which medical interventions and experiments have gotten increasingly out of control. Political and legal attempts to control the spread of cloning by Presidents Bill Clinton and George W. Bush are simply further evidence for many that the brave-new-world fiction of George Orwell could become a reality. People are anxious that a world of secret medical experimentation is already upon us. The globalization of disease, the reproduction of people by means of new technologies, the degradation of the environment, the spread of cyborgs, and the mechanization of the domestic environment have in turn given rise to speculation about the postmodernization of the human body, which would be a hybrid phenomenon, precariously poised among nature, technology, and culture. In postmodern theory, human beings will no longer be metaphorically mechanical; they will in fact be mechanized. I have already argued that these dystopian visions of human beings and the transformation of their bodies are exaggerated. Such technical devices may become available to the very rich, but they are unlikely to have a major impact on the majority of the population. We do, however, have to take seriously the general impact of technology on health and illness. For example, the World Health Organization (WHO) estimates that 1.2 million people are killed annually in road accidents, and by 2020 traffic accidents will kill more people each year than HIV, diarrhea, or tuberculosis. The mechanization of travel and the development of societies based on "automobility" do have major consequences for health that were not envisioned by the early public health movement. The globalization of disease and the notion of automobility can be usefully illustrated by the outbreak of SARS in January 2003 in the Chinese province of Guangdong. SARS is a unique form of pneumonia that is caused by an influenza-type virus rather than bacteria. WHO warned that SARS was moving across the world with "the speed of a jet." By early April 2003, there were 1,268 reported cases and 61 deaths in Hong Kong. Having infected hundreds of people in China and Vietnam, the syndrome spread quickly to the United States and Europe, carried mainly by air passengers exiting Asia through Singapore and Hong Kong. SARS had a major impact on the Asian economy and led many air carriers in the region, such as Qantas, to cancel flights as governments warned their citizens not to fly. SARS is a clear illustration of the unintended health consequences of globalization.

CONCLUSION: GLOBALIZATION AND MEDICAL PLURALISM

Complementary and alternative medicine (CAM) is part of the broader social movements that are concerned with consumer choice, holistic healing, feminism, self-help, and the environment (A. Scott 1998). These social transformations are indicated by changes in medical terminology. What used to be the dubious practice of "alternative medicine" eventually became "complementary medicine" and more recently "integrated medicine" or "holistic medicine." One important and problematic question is whether the growing acceptance of CAM is mainstreaming, co-opting, or neutralizing. What is evident, however, is that the growth of CAM represents a major transformation of the relationships between doctors and their patients and between doctors and the larger scientific community.

We have seen that from 1910 to 1970, scientific medicine enjoyed a golden age of increasing influence, status, and wealth. The research hospitals were models of scientific application, acute diseases that had ravaged Western societies were being eliminated, and the medical profession enjoyed the trust and respect of middle-class society. Flexner's assumptions laid the foundation for the medical model of illness, established the social conditions for medical dominance, and produced the professional circumstances that underpinned the patient's role.

The doctor's clinical authority was unchallenged, and the patient was expected to be docile and compliant. In the United States, physicians working in a private health-care environment were able to establish and control the nature of medical care and the circumstances in which it was delivered. The American Medical Association and the British Medical Association were powerful professional lobbies that exercised significant political power on behalf of medical science through Congress and Parliament. The professions had considerable success in claiming that collectivist innovations in the delivery of health care would undermine the principles of individualism, self-help, and self-reliance, on which Western medicine had been built. However, the end of the "golden age of doctoring" (McKinlay and Marceau 1998) was signaled by Richard Nixon's 1970 speech announcing the crisis in health care in the United States. The health crisis was an economic crisis brought about by the graying population, increasing problems with chronic illness, rising insurance costs, and the expense of medical technology. It was also a professional crisis, as the traditional authority and autonomy of doctors were eroded by corporate control of doctoring, declining trust in doctors, and growing demand for different types of medicine, such as CAM.

The social and political conditions that produced professional medicine have changed for a variety of reasons. While allopathic medicine has provided spectacular cures for acute illness, chronic illness that is related to lifestyle, sedentary occupations, and an aging population cannot be easily cured or effectively treated. Medical science appears to have experienced a number of limitations in the effective treatment of cancer, heart disease, diabetes, and other degenerative conditions for which germ theory—the basis of the medical model—does not offer easy or efficient solutions. A public that has become increasingly sophisticated and conscious of its rights as health consumers has flocked to acupuncture, aromatherapy, yoga, homeopathy, and chiropractic.

The dissatisfaction of patients with intrusive care by conventional medicine is an important factor in the growing support for CAM. The limitations of invasive measures in the treatment of cancer have, in particular, stimulated the quest for alternative systems of treatment. Although mainstream medical science has accepted research indicating that diet and lifestyle are significant in the etiology of certain cancers, physicians have been relatively slow to recognize the role of diet in the treatment of patients. In the United States, however, partly through the influence of such scientists as Linus Pauling, research centers, including the M. D. Anderson Cancer Center in Texas, have examined the contribution of nutrition in the treatment of childhood cancers. The argument is not that nutritional regimes can replace chemotherapy but that nutritional management is complementary to existing medical technologies. Although there may be valid skepticism of the efficacy of CAM responses to cancer, survival rates with existing conventional treatments remain depressingly low. In the United Kingdom, which is at the bottom of the European nations, health expenditure as a percentage of gross domestic product was 6.9 percent in the late 1990s, and five-year survival rates for colon and breast cancer were 36 percent and 63 percent. The corresponding figures for the United States were 12.7 percent of gross domestic product and 60 percent and 82 percent. One conclusion is that consumer demand for a wider range of choice in the management of cancers has produced better treatment regimes and outcomes.

Consumer lobby groups focusing on women's health have also had important consequences for health care, but the management of pregnancy remains a controversial issue. In the United States, the women's health movement gathered momentum in the early 1970s, and Barbara Ehrenreich and Deirdre English's *For Her Own Good* (1978) became a classic in feminist critical theory, but the advances in patient empowerment have been uneven. Disillusioned by the increasing dependence on cesarean section, women have demanded the services of midwives and more supportive environments in the hospital. Although few women now deliver at home with the assistance of a midwife, hospitals have developed birthing rooms, which resemble conventional domestic rooms, as an alternative to the impersonal and alienating environment of a conventional delivery ward, which depends on extensive technology and resembles a laboratory. In addition, greater attention is being paid to the importance of bonding between mother and child after birth. At the same time, rates of cesarean deliveries remain high, and many cesareans are thought to be unnecessary. In the United States, cesarean sections had risen to 21.2 percent of all births by 1994. Despite years of criticism, cesarean sections in England and Wales have risen sevenfold in the last thirty years, and in 2001 cesarean delivery accounted for one in five births. Approximately 60 percent of those deliveries were classified as emergencies, but 7 percent were performed for no specific medical reason. While the rising number of older women who are becoming mothers and the threat of litigation can explain some of the increase, social pref-

erences also play a part. Cesarean sections are thought to be
safer, easier, and less painful, and elective cesareans have become fashionable as such celebrities as Victoria Beckham, Eliz-
abeth Hurley, and Patsy Kensit have promoted the aesthetic
advantages of the procedure. The irony is that given the short-
age of qualified midwives, obstetricians are more likely to opt
for cesarean delivery whenever a complication presents itself.

In general terms, patients' rights and consumer demand
have pressured health-care professionals to provide more holistic care. In the United States, the slow but significant growth
of health-care insurance for alternative medicine and the growing number of young doctors who do not join the American
Medical Association have been regarded by some sociologists as
an erosion of medical dominance (Pescosolido and Boyer 2001,
183). The medical profession has also changed under the impact of technical advances in medicine, making for commercial
transformations of medical practice. We need to consider these
changes within the framework of the sociology of the professions. The legitimacy of the medical profession rests not only
on its political power but also on the trust of the public. The
two dimensions of professionalism are medical dominance and
the consulting ethic, with the first requiring the support of the
state and the second depending on public confidence and trust.
These two dimensions have been transformed by the growth of
corporate and global medical systems. Recent corporate developments in capturing the commercial potential of health and
illness constitute the global emergence of the medical economy.
These global changes are not only transforming the traditional
doctor-patient relationship, but they are also opening up possibilities, the directions of which are unclear.

In terms of the growth of public confidence and trust in the medical profession, a variety of technical inventions and discoveries of nineteenth-century medicine—such as immunization—established the scientific authority of medicine as a profession. For the lay public, improvements in survival rates from surgery have been especially visible evidence of the scientific basis of contemporary medical practice. The effectiveness of twentieth-century surgery was consolidated through improvements in anaesthesia, electrolyte physiology, and cardiopulmonary physiology. Although the quality of general practice still depends in large measure on interpersonal skills that can be fully acquired only through experience rather than training, the status of medical institutions in society depends significantly on "hard" science and technology. Medical technology presents simultaneously and paradoxically the promise of significant therapeutic improvements in the management of illness and significant risks to the well-being and comfort of patients.

Professional medicine has long been concerned with regulating, largely unsuccessfully, self-medication and "folk medicine" (Baks 1991), but in a high-risk environment it is also important to control scientific medicine. In order to gain the full benefits of medical innovation, there has to be some regulation of the social and cultural risks associated with contemporary medical sciences in relation to cloning, new reproductive technologies, organ transplants, surgical intervention for fetal abnormalities, cosmetic surgery, the prescription of antidepressants, sex selection of children, or more recently, cryonically frozen patients. Who should exercise these regulatory constraints or governance over the medical sciences? In Britain, the British Medical Association has been criticized for its failure to monitor effectively doctors who have been charged with criminal offenses or malpractice. The nadir of trust in doctor-patient relations in Britain in recent history may have been reached by the revelations surrounding the medical practice of Harold Shipman, who in the latter part of his career killed over a hundred elderly patients in his care. The apparent instability and contradictions in the expert advice surrounding the foot-and-mouth epidemic of 2001 further eroded the authority of scientific or expert opinion in Britain. Lay confidence in science and the food chain has been further battered by a 20 percent to 30 percent rise in Creutzfeldt-Jakob disease (CJD) in Britain in recent years. These examples suggest that the tensions between public trust, uninsurable risk and scientific legitimacy have generally undermined confidence in expert systems (Beck 1992; Giddens 1990), and as a result the public has experimented with alternative and less intrusive healing systems.

Any sociological understanding of medicine in contemporary society will have to examine the economics of the corporate structure of medical practice and will have to locate that corporate structure within a framework of global commercial and cultural processes. The deregulation of global markets as a result of the neoliberal policies of the 1970s has had the unintended consequence of bringing about the globalization of disease. The return of the "old" infectious diseases—TB, malaria, typhoid, and cholera—will not only have significant negative consequences for the economies of the developing world but will also reappear in the affluent West as a consequence of the globalization of transportation, tourism, and labor markets. It is unlikely that corporations will adopt policies of corporate citizenship quickly or effectively enough to exercise constraint and to institutionalize environmental audits to regulate their impact on local communities, but these global developments have created new opportunities for the exercise of consumer power as a mechanism whereby the negative impact of corporate enterprise on fragile communities and environments can be challenged. Developments in health care must be firmly connected to existing debates about civil society and human rights. Health—along with employment, education, and welfare—is a fundamental entitlement of citizenship, but this entitlement is often difficult to implement in a world economy in which risks are global. The question of health as entitlement raises difficult political and policy questions because there is an inevitable tension between citizenship as a bundle of national rights and obligations and human rights as a system of entitlement that does not rest directly on the sovereignty of particular nation-states.

The growth of corporate control over medical care has contributed to the decline of professional autonomy, initiative, and social status. The neoconservative emphasis on the free market and aggressive entrepreneurship has brought about a decline in the social status of general practitioners by converting them to the hired employees of profit-making, private-sector health systems. The professional physician who is hired by a commercial enterprise has to make a profit in addition to providing an adequate system of health care. Furthermore, the contemporary development of health care in the United States has brought about a new emphasis on medical specialization that has undermined, or at least threatened, the occupational coherence and solidarity of medicine as a professional group. In addition to this internal division, with the growth of consumer groups, malpractice legislation, and public alarm with technological medicine, there has been a renewed interest in more holistic medical services through alternative and complementary systems. The commercialization of medicine and the dominance of free-market principles have had the paradoxical consequence of eroding the foundations of the traditional, autonomous professional physician as an individual provider of care in a direct relationship with the client.

While neoconservative policies may have changed the conditions under which the traditional autonomy of the medical profession was sustained, they have also had serious consequences for consumers. These consequences have become apparent in a variety of areas of welfare. In the United States, for example, poverty among children has increased by 30 percent since 1979. Between 1981 and 1982, eleven states showed increases in the infant mortality rate, as well as considerable differences between black and white mortality rates. In Michigan, for example, infant mortality rates rose for the first time in more than thirty years, to more than thirteen per one thousand live births. The rising infant mortality rate is associated with an increase in poverty and unemployment, a decline in nutrition, and the loss of health insurance coverage through the new limits on Medicaid. Nixon's health-care crisis was manifest in a rising number of uninsured Americans, an increasing use of alternative medicine, the inability of germ theory to contribute to the treatment of chronic illness, and the growth of self-help movements. While there are significant indicators of increasing poverty, the private health sector has enjoyed buoyant profitability and expansion. The economic and political importance of the tax cuts under the administration of Ronald Reagan was that by reducing revenue to the state, they curtailed the ability of future governments to introduce new social welfare programs to ease hardship, stimulate employment schemes, and restore welfare measures. As medicine has become increasingly specialized, the general practitioner has become the conduit to specialized medical care, referring the patient to specialists further on in the chain of care. The commercialization of services and the increasing anonymity of medical practitioners in relation to their patients have eroded the relations of trust that traditionally characterized medical practice. Patients have turned to self-help partly because they cannot afford allopathic medicine and partly because they distrust invasive medication and treatment.

Of course, anxiety about the pace of technology and its pernicious consequences has been a feature of public inquiry into medicine for a considerable time. In the postwar period, doctors, especially in research hospitals, were criticized as "priests of the machine," and in the doctor-patient relationship it was feared that medical technology would create "physician-centered medicine" rather than "patient-centered medicine." Scientific anxieties about "medical harm" and adverse drug reactions began to appear in the medical literature in the 1950s and 1960s. The negative effects of the drug Prozac became a particular issue in public awareness of medical harm in America (Kramer 1994). With the expansion of the legal rights of patients, trust between patients and their doctors has been tested by the emergence of a culture of litigation. Medical-malpractice litigation has become an important aspect of modern legal practice, and lack of confidence in medical practice has become a contentious arena in public life. At the same time, the technical and technological problems of medicine have become global, and the risks of medical failure or mismanagement have massive legal and economic consequences for the health-care system.

The development of new reproductive technologies, genetic engineering, and the enhancement of human traits point toward a "second" medical revolution, one that combines microbiology and informational science. This revolution is seen to present a major challenge to traditional institutions and religious cosmologies, but it may also present a threat to the processes of political governance. The modern notion of a risk society provokes questions about the unintended consequences of medical change, whether the technological imperative can be regulated, and the relationships between pure research, commercialization, and academic autonomy. For example, pharmaceutical companies have turned to contract research organizations (CROs) rather than universities to undertake basic research on drugs. CROs are cheaper and less independent than academic institutions. In the United States, about 60 percent of industry-based pharmaceutical grants have gone to CROs rather than universities. The academic community has argued that such research is not systematically published and is unlikely to be critical of the pharmaceutical products. In short, such "private" forms of research are not compatible with the public norms of publication, debate, and criticism that are assumed to be essential to scientific objectivity. Because the pharmaceutical industry is currently dominated by a limited number of corporations—ICI, Ciba, and Hoechst—there are serious problems with respect to the regulation of the industry and the freedom of market relations.

Medical institutions and professions are subject to global pressures, especially from competitive insurance and funding arrangements. To take one obvious illustration, the ownership and the current development of the pharmaceutical industry are global arrangements. Health-care systems are also on the verge of dependence on global electronic communications. One remarkable example is telesurgery, which involves the use of robot-assisted distance surgery. The techniques were pioneered by the U.S. military to provide expert medical service in the field, but they could also make a valuable contribution to aid workers in developing societies and provide important training for young surgeons. Health-care systems are often slow to adopt innovations in information technology, however, because the hardware and software are thought to be insufficiently advanced to make useful contributions. Nonetheless, it is assumed that in the future, patients and doctors will use broadband technologies to deliver health-care packages to homes and hospitals. The growth of e-health will create virtual hospitals, transform health education, deliver health services to patients who have limited mobility, and improve health delivery to remote communities. The technology and delivery systems for such innovations will necessarily be global, and they will be organized and owned by global health corporations.

Although the dominant trend of much recent medical sociology has been to emphasize the negative effects of globalization and to regard e-health as a further commodification of medicine, alternative trends indicate a growth in consumer autonomy, increased involvement of patient groups in decision making, and an erosion of medical dominance in favor of "bottom-up" participation. For a variety of specific conditions and diseases, patients have increased their use of consumer Web sites for care, support, and information. To some extent, the model of the consumer/patient lobby group has been provided by the HIV/AIDS epidemic, in response to which activists have successfully challenged medical control and shaped the nature of AIDS research and research funding. AIDS Web sites have played an important global part in organizing such consumer movements to improve health care (Altman 2001). A variety of social movements—the human rights, women's, environmental, labor, peace, and religious movements—have exploited the opportunities of electronic network communication. Electronic networks also open up opportunities for lay health groups. Cystic fibrosis (CF) provides a particularly good example. As the life expectancy of its sufferers has increased to around thirty years of age, public health-care systems have had to rely increasingly on home help and lay caregivers. There are now ranges of CF Web sites that provide health information, such as instructions on the use of intravenous injections for home care. The result is the sidelining of professional medical control and the transformation of the nature of medical authority.

With the increase in chronic illness as a result of HIV/AIDS, aging, and changes in lifestyle, the management of care may pass more and more into lay hands supported by e-health systems. Obviously, this is a mixed blessing, as more care will devolve to female heads of households, but it does represent an increase in lay power. Of course, corporate e-health will take a predatory interest in "nativistic," or "indigenous," pharmacy and will seek to commercialize alternative health care and to monopolize medical knowledge and research. We may envisage an endlessly circular struggle involving centralized and localized e-health and corporate and lay interests. The growth of CAM will clearly be assisted by global information systems that work at a local level, because patients will be selecting health-care alternatives directly from Web sites.

Foucault's historical work on the birth of the clinic demonstrates the intimate connections between the French Revolution, the growth of anatomy, and the transformation of the concept of disease. Today we are going through a revolution of equal magnitude. The twentieth-century monopoly of mainstream health care and health provision that was enjoyed by professional medicine and the dominance of allopathic science have been shaken by a complex set of global processes: new technologies, changes in consumer demand, the globalization of medical systems, the differentiation and fragmentation of scientific knowledge, the transformation of the pattern of disease, and a variety of new social movements. New configurations of power are producing new systems of knowledge, within which CAM will come to play an important, but probably unpredictable, part. The global revolution in health care will in turn compel the scientific community to reconsider and redefine the purposes of medicine.

Chapter 4
TIME, SELF, AND DISRUPTION

INTRODUCTION: NARRATIVES OF THE ILLNESS EXPERIENCE

CONFLICT IN DOCTOR-PATIENT INTERACTION has been an enduring topic of medical sociology, partly as a critical response to the presumption of social consensus in Talcott Parsons's conception of the sick role (1951). Different concepts of time are central to disagreements and implicit conflicts between doctors and patients. The effective allocation of patients in the organization of time is a routine source of tension and conflict in the management of hospitals. For economists, time is money because it is a limited resource over which there are social conflicts. In organizational terms, time is a scarce resource, but we also need to pay attention to the social meaning of time.

Disagreements and conflicts over the meaning of time are frequent in doctor-patient interactions because patients, especially those with chronic conditions, tend to calculate their recovery time in a manner that is typically inconsistent with medical models of the normal progression of disease. While time as a topic has been somewhat neglected in mainstream sociology, in medical sociology Barney Glaser and Anselm Strauss (1968a) have provided an important insight into the temporal dimensions of social interaction. Strauss's legacy of grounded theory provides the foundation of a typology of the temporal character of disease, the timing of sickness in the patient's life cycle, and the position of the patient in his or her life course. This chapter demonstrates how the typology can illuminate tensions between the subjective experience of time by the patient and professional time, or "clock time." Clearly, patients and professionals give a priority to time as a scarce resource, where the timeliness or untimeliness of disease has conflicting meanings. Priorities in the social allocation of resources reflect differences in social values and create hierarchies of expectation. Priorities of values organize scarce resources and constitute moral schedules or queues that significantly affect the treatment of patients, especially geriatric patients.

In this chapter, we will explore illness as a disruption in the temporal structure of everyday life and examine the role of narratives of the patient's illness experience. The disruptions of chronic illness have serious implications for maintaining a sense of self-continuity and normality. Narratives help patients with chronic illness to sustain a commitment to the future and to the possibility of remission or recovery, and hence "narratives of restitution" have an important place in therapy (A. W. Frank 1995, 1991a). While doctors and patients conspire to maintain positive narratives of recovery, they typically subscribe to different interpretations of events within the narrative. Expectations about time, remission, recovery, and health are not necessarily shared or described in the same narratives. Sociological research has demonstrated important differences between clock time and subjective time in medical institutions and has found that doctors' perceptions and patients' experiences of illness are often incompatible (Pierret 2003). The study of time as a resource of social action also raises general issues about the management of scarcity in social life. Queues are an obvious illustration of temporal scarcity in everyday life, but they play an important part in the bureaucratic management of clinics and hospitals.

TIME AND SELF: THE LEGACY OF GROUNDED THEORY

While symbolic interactionism dominated empirical research in medical sociology in the 1960s and early 1970s, more recent approaches have been influenced by social constructionism, the poststructuralism of Foucault, and postmodernism. In a comprehensive review of the field, Ken Plummer (2000, 205) lamented the neglect of symbolic interactionism in terms of its contributions to the study of identity, the body, and habitus in recent writing about intimacy, subjectivity, and embodiment. The irony is that these new approaches, especially the notion that the social world is socially constructed, are compatible with, or were developed by, symbolic interactionism. A core assumption of symbolic interactionism is that social actors continuously negotiate the social world and the everyday world is consequently produced by their collective strategies. Time is an important dimension of this negotiated order. More important for medical sociology, time has to be understood in the context of the experience of illness by people who are passing through the life cycle both individually and collectively.

In this introductory discussion, I shall concentrate on the contributions of Anselm L. Strauss and Barney G. Glaser to medical sociology. The tradition of micro-empirical research in Straussian medical sociology eventually gave rise to the grounded-theory tradition. Glaser and Strauss (1968b) distinguished between formal and substantive theory. Formal theory refers to any conceptual area of sociology, whereas grounded theory applies to any substantive field, such as education or medicine. Grounded theory involves a general method of comparative research in which theory is discovered through inductively exploring research findings. Grounded theory was associated with the use of qualitative methods in social research, in which generating theory is the principal aim of the researcher (Strauss and Corbin 1997). The word *grounded* refers to the fact that Strauss's theoretical ideas came directly from his empirical observations and were consequently grounded in his rich research data. Strauss's grounded theory was inductive, cumulative, and middle range. He made major contributions to the study of professions, medical organizations, and the experience of dying. In approaching Straussian grounded theory as an example of symbolic interactionism, we can note that interactionism is organized according to three themes: settings, processes, and identities. Within each of these categories, time is a social resource and the product of negotiation.

The symbolic-interactionist view of the social world as a negotiated order characterized the whole of Strauss's approach, from his early essays on "The Hospital and Its Negotiated Order" (Strauss et al. 1963) to his later work in *Negotiations* (1978). Society is something that is continuously produced by endless micronegotiations for resources, identity, and meaning. Strauss studied the negotiation of workplace settings such as hospitals, specifically looking at the way the social interconnections of technology, work organization, and occupational clusters are resolved or managed (Strauss et al. 1985). Hospitals are bureaucratic clusters of work sites through which patients pass in a more or less continuous flow. The passage of patients becomes increasingly contingent, partly because the complexity of medical technology has fragmented chronic illness and dispersed patients across many work teams.

The idea that settings are negotiated was not of course unique to Strauss. Much of the impetus for such a view of social reality came from Erving Goffman, especially in *Asylums* (1961), which holds that the structure of social interactions involves constant negotiations between front- and backstage settings. Another illustration relevant to medical sociology is the work of Julius Roth on the career of TB patients in a sanatorium (1963, 1984). In *Timetables,* Roth (1963) studied how conflicts between patients and physicians are negotiated in hospitals and how contradictions between professional and lay expectations about time are resolved. Patients regarded timely release from an institution as a measure of getting better, but such lay definitions of improvement do not necessarily correspond to the time schedules of doctors. Another illustration might be taken from David Sudnow's study of the social organization of dying, in which the management of dead patients and the ritual order of the mortuary have specific temporal structures (1967). Yet another classic of this epoch is Fred Davis's study of polio victims and their families in a temporal "passage through crisis" (1963).

These studies show the dominant impact of symbolic interactionism on American medical sociology in the 1960s. The linking theme of these studies is the idea that medical work is no different from other forms of work. As such, it has to take place in institutional settings, where there must be some negotiation of scarce resources. Negotiations occur in hospital settings in order to get things accomplished despite conflicts over resources and the meanings of social interaction (Strauss 1978). Perhaps another characteristic of symbolic interactionism is its irreverent tone toward medical practices. Interactionist research demystified hospital settings and showed that physicians, like other workers, are subject to the vagaries of interaction settings, including endless negotiations (H. S. Becker et al. 1961).

In his final work, Strauss came to argue that these settings of action should be thought of as "continual permutations of action." Within this framework, he spoke of "the conditional matrix" and the conditional paths of action through it. The social realm is a series of circles from the global to the setting of action itself, and the task of sociology is to chart the pathways of action through such conditional matrices. The paths through such social circles can be "short, long, thick, thin, loose, tight, startling, commonplace, visible, invisible" (1993, 60). The analysis of these pathways from the everyday to the global demonstrates that the micro-macro distinction between the everyday and the global arena is untenable.

Strauss remains influential in contemporary sociology through his analysis of trajectories, in which social relations are a series of transformations of biography through distinctive status passages. Individuals mature by going through definite and specific stages in life that transform their status, or standing, in the community. These concepts were elaborated on in a collection of influential empirical studies of death and dying (Glaser and Strauss 1965, 1968a, 1971). While the course of an illness forms a pattern that is recognized by doctors and nurses who chart the development of disease through various stages, *trajectory* refers "not only to the physiological unfolding of a patient's disease but to the total *organization of work* done over that course, plus the *impact* on those involved with that work and its organization" (Strauss et al. 1985, 8). Different conditions or diseases have different trajectories insofar as they involve or require different forms of expressive and instrumental work. The trajectory of throat cancer is very different from that of prostate cancer because the latter is often slow and prolonged and the early symptoms may not be obvious to the individual. Throat cancers are more rapid and invasive, and their impact on speech has an immediate consequence for social interaction. In this sense, trajectory is about disease management. Disease is not an individual with a condition who is passing through time but an individual with a condition who is a member of a social team coping with contingencies in a negotiated medical setting.

For example, dying is a form of status passage, and thus it is a social process guided by social expectations of appropriate behavior. These expectations constitute a set of "dying trajectories" that organize normal and abnormal situations. A lingering dying trajectory is described in the case study published as *Anguish* (Glaser and Strauss 1970). The trajectories involve the medical staff's expectations that a patient is dying, that the process will have a particular duration, and that it will therefore have a specific temporal shape. By establishing a social organization of dying, these norms and practices give some institutional order to dying, thereby avoiding the disruptive and contingent events that would otherwise undermine the smooth running of a hospital.

Studies of dying trajectories gave rise to a rich terminology—including *coping strategies, identity dilemmas, extended-birthing trajectories, hospital biography,* and *identity loss*—that is concerned with the temporal structure of identities and organizations. Indeed, it was argued that "an organization can be conceived as a temporal matrix" (Strauss et al. 1985, 280) because it is constituted by the temporal dimensions of occupational groups, work schedules, and patient biographies. Organizations involve the management of timetables.

Social interactionism has approached identity as a social definition that is unstable, negotiated in social settings, open to dispute and challenge, and managed through a range of status passages. In *Mirrors and Masks,* Strauss (1959) used metaphors to show that identity is both a presentation of a range of masks for public inspection and a set of mirrors within which the individual self-reflexively contemplates identity. While many status passages are relatively formal and predictable, many others are not. Disease as a status passage is important for self-identity because its onset is often unexpected and its consequences can be devastating for the individual, because in essence they involve the loss of normal activities, social relations, self-confidence, and security. Diseases typically involve uncertainty and risk and have major but unpredictable consequences for social relations and self-identity. Patients may require considerable "coaching" if they are to pass through these crises successfully. While key events in the life course can be anticipated, the disruptions of illness and their effects on identity are difficult to predict, particularly in the case of acute illness and accident. Straussian paradigms for the study of the consequences of illness on self-identity have had an important impact on the sociological imagination. Many of these contributions to the study of illness, time, and identity have been collected in *Grounded Theory in Practice* (Strauss and Corbin

1997), and the research of Kathy Charmaz (1994) on chronically ill men and of Celia Orona (1990) on Alzheimer's disease has been particularly important. Both contributions are concerned with the sociological understanding of identity change in the chronically ill.

Because Strauss was concerned with the sociology of work and organizations, the body did not play a prominent role in his early research. Toward the end of his life, however, he turned more explicitly to the interactions among body, disease, and trajectory. The body biography was an important framework in Juliet Corbin and Strauss's *Unending Work and Care* (1988). The key idea in this work is that illness trajectories have a particular shape, and to understand the shape of a trajectory, we need to consider the interrelationships. Bodies and biographies unfold along two intertwined trajectories—the "body-biography chain"—that are set within a conditional matrix. Thus, a heart attack affects home and work and transforms the anticipated or normal biographical trajectory, which is also dependent on social class, regional location, and available medical help. Many illness experiences do not have a simple impact; instead, they disrupt the trajectory of the body biography, which has, in effect, no coherent shape or pattern. The body-biography trajectory may assume many different forms or shapes. Acute and chronic conditions have very different temporal structures, and the interaction between body and biography depends on a range of sociostructural factors (Corbin and Strauss 1987). Other elements play a role, too: identities are multiple; the illness trajectory converts the patient into a case—for example, a cardiac failure; and the classificatory scheme of the disease itself modifies the shape of the trajectory (Star and Bowker 1997).

The symbolic-interaction tradition is important as a paradigm for thinking about time and disease. It invites us to combine the existential issue of the timeliness of acute and chronic illness with an analysis of the structures of the life course, aging, and generations. It connects our experience of personal troubles to their institutional settings, explores the pervasive contradictions between our experiences and their public significance, and considers how these contradictions are negotiated. Strauss has provided us with a profound grasp of the negotiation of the social order as a precarious set of arrangements for coping with the world.

The problem of time has also been an important part of modern philosophy (Heidegger 1958). However, philosophical speculation has been relatively weak in its treatment of the contingencies of the everyday world and the need to negotiate the social order through an endless struggle over material and cultural resources. The social order has a temporality that must be managed by the social actors involved. These social actors are also shot through with temporalities, however. The social order is an effect of the negotiation that takes place over different orders of temporality.

TIME AND DISEASE

The tradition of symbolic interactionism, particularly the legacy of Strauss, raises questions about the timeliness or untimeliness of disease and sickness episodes. This discussion can be usefully framed in terms of the sociology of the sick role (Parsons 1951, 1999a). In his analysis of the social dimension of being sick, Talcott Parsons argued that sickness is a social role, legitimated by conformity to a medical regime, whereby the patient could acquire temporary release from normal duties, such as paid employment. The question of time was important to Parsons's theory of the sick-role concept, but his model is open to the criticism that it cannot provide a satisfactory account of the differences between acute and chronic illness. The symbolic-interactionist tradition of Goffman, Davis, and Roth responded critically to Parsons because the sick-role concept does not adequately recognize conflicts in doctor-patient encounters. From this critical debate, the sociology of the "experience of illness" (Conrad and Bury 1997, 374) was an important alternative to Parsons's approach. The patient's experience of illness and medical interpretations of the patient's condition are often disconnected, unrelated, and contradictory. In particular, the sick-role concept is inappropriate as an approach to chronic illness. Whereas acute illness is the implicit core of the sick-role concept, Straussian sociology examined how people attempt to live normal lives while coping with chronic illness and how their experiences affect their family and friends. Strauss and Glaser's *Chronic Illness and the Quality of Life* (1975) mapped out the principal coordinates of what became an established tradition of research on chronicity and its impact on the normal routines of everyday life. Through this research tradition on the clash of perspectives between lay sufferers and their professional caregivers, studies of time and sickness began to describe an important analytic topic on the timeliness of sickness and disease.

While there is plenty of research on conflicts over knowledge in the doctor-patient relationship (Turner 1995a, 39–46), disagreements about time have been less prominent in sociology, with the obvious exception of Roth's work on hospital timetables. We can initially describe a model that identifies four temporal dimensions of sickness. The first of these is the temporal shape of disease and sickness in terms of their probable internal rhythms. Diseases and conditions have their own rhythm and momentum. We use metaphors to describe the speed and shape of a disease that comes eventually to a climax and a conclusion, such as the death of the patient. For example, fevers are said to be galloping, but the chronicity of diabetes typically expresses itself as a slow progression. Tuberculosis is a wasting disease. Although medical interventions can often delay or modify their progress, diseases have different temporal structures and velocities. The second dimension is the clock time of professional work practices in medical settings and the bureaucratic management of patients as cases in a numerical sequence. A hospital is an organization that attempts to regulate the flow of cases to match its own resources. Third, are the shared social assumptions about the appropriate timing of a disease within the typical life cycle of the patient in general. Finally, there is the subjective definition of the timing of a disease event from the perspective of the patient—the experience of illness.

The literature on chronicity (Roth and Conrad 1987) suggests that there are important areas of disagreement between lay and professional assessments of the proper timing of and time for a sickness event. Like other resources, time has to be socially negotiated. Thomas Mann's *Magic Mountain* is a brilliant fictional exploration of the complexities of conflicting assumptions of time, whereby, in many respects, the TB sanatorium exists outside time. To take their cure, the TB patients in Mann's novel are secluded in an alpine resort, where social life and the temporal demands of a normal existence are brought to a halt. They live in a social hiatus. They are locked into their disease just as they are locked out of society. The novel provides a poignant account of their struggle to make sense of their time out of society and their conflicts with the medical hierarchy.

The sociological literature provides ample evidence of the differences between patient and professional time; the management of a regular and predictable flow of deliveries within a maternity unit through the inducement of births is an example. The sequencing of events within a hospital setting forms a "moral queue" as the events are determined by social, not natural, arrangements. Within any social group, there will be assumptions and expectations about the appropriateness of disease and death within the life cycle of individuals. Such lay beliefs will clearly include popular versions of professional opinion. It is commonly said that pneumonia, for example, is an old man's friend and that death from pneumonia can be a timely event for the elderly. In Britain, for example, where euthanasia is not legally or routinely available, elderly patients are sometimes subjected to medical interventions to extend their lives against their wishes.

The timing of a disease needs to be considered within the life span of the individual and the cohort or generation of which he or she is a part. While prostate cancer for older men or breast cancer for older women might be timely occurrences within the life cycle, cancer in children is an untimely event that requires pervasive intervention. Because a death in childhood is tragic, it demands a great deal of social effort on the part of doctors, nurses, and auxiliary staff to make sense of the event. The death of a child is an affront to our assumptions about time and meaning.

Because there are fundamental social assumptions about the distribution and timing of disease and sickness, it is important to consider queuing in social life. Normal queues, for example at a bus stop or a bank, are methods of organizing scarce resources in a system that distributes goods and services in a relatively fair and predictable manner. Normal queues are matters of convenience, with the first to arrive getting served first. A moral queue is a method of allocation in terms of social values rather than convenience. Putting women and children in lifeboats when a ship is sinking is a queuing mechanism in which moral judgments about vulnerability are paramount. Moral queues are social facts in terms of Durkheim's rules of sociological method. As an individual, I may hold serious doubts about the principle of women and children first, but there is considerable collective agreement about the underlying values of queues as a component of the social structure. Moral queues reflect general social values in a society and in medicine informally prioritize patients in terms of their moral worth and their vulnerability.

Jumping queues may elicit a strong sense of shame. There are contradictions, however, between the economics and the morality of scarce resources. Recent public outrage in Britain about allegations that doctors issue do-not-resuscitate (DNR) orders for elderly patients without their knowledge or the consent of their families illustrates the conflict between economic rationality and moral standards. Medical authorities who are confronted by scarce resources will experience tensions between normal and moral queues. In Britain, voluntary groups that provide services to the elderly—such as Age Concern—have sponsored research showing that ageism is an implicit prejudice that allocates treatment in emergency units in favor of young people. There is some suspicion that alcoholics, members of minority groups, down-and-outs, and HIV-positive patients are also more likely to receive a DNR notice or its equivalent than are members of the public who are perceived to be upstanding citizens. In any case, the division between public hospitals, which are underfunded, and private hospitals, which are commercial operations, involves a stratification of patients according to those who can pay and those who cannot. In the popular press, inequality in treatment is often regarded as an example of racism or ageism, but in fact it displays different queuing principles. In the modern hospital, conflicts over scarcity and the meaning of time for doctors and their clients are inevitable. The essence of the conflict is that for the patient, time is ontologically scarce; for a rational bureaucracy, time is economically scarce.

Finally, the subjective time of patients is also problematic. Sociological studies of aging have discovered a tension between the subjective definition of time and the objective chronology of people getting older (Featherstone and Wernick 1995). This tension is often expressed in terms of the "inner body," which remains young and ageless, and an "outer body," which is obviously subject to decline and aging. As we get older, the tension between our inner self and our outer image becomes more acute and disconnected. In a consumer society, especially among the affluent middle classes, the tension between objective and subjective body times has been exacerbated by consumer images of perpetual youthfulness, and hence medical science is increasingly expected to produce commercially lucrative answers for aging bodies. There is also a generational effect. The postwar baby boomers still occupy many of the leading positions in the social structure and were socialized in a culture of permanent youthfulness (Edmunds and Turner 2002). This generation continues to have an important impact on popular and professional values regarding the life cycle. Celebrity geriatric rock stars are expected to defy aging through cosmetic surgery, transplants, implants, skin treatment, diet, and exercise.

These social norms imply that conditions that curtail the full enjoyment of an active life are by definition untimely. While some forms of chronic illness, such as rheumatoid arthritis, are common in old age, they are often rejected by those who suffer from the condition as incompatible with self-definitions of time and the life course (G. Williams 1984). The emphasis on youthfulness in modern societies has eroded social support for the notion that there are definite stages within the life course that are necessary and unavoidable, such as menopause in women or impotence in men. The idea that there is a midlife crisis is generally contested. Because the inner, subjective time of the individual is resistant to the vagaries of an aging body, social roles do not provide a comfortable transition from paid work to retirement and inactivity. In the history of the sociology of aging, the critical response to disengagement theory and the current emphasis on activity theory are barometers of social change. It had been assumed that successful aging requires a slow but steady withdrawal or disengagement from social roles (Cumming 1963; Cumming and Henry 1961). The end of reproduction, menopause, retirement, and withdrawal from community responsibilities were regarded as normal stages in a gradual process of aging and maturity. These assumptions were later challenged by activity theory, which claims that the real problem with aging is isolation and loneliness and therefore disengagement theory represents an image of aging that in modern society is too passive (Atchley 1989).

Only when the four dimensions—disease time, bureaucratic clock time, the social life cycle, and subjective time—coincide can one speak about a sickness or disease episode being timely. The transformation of life-cycle norms and the assumption that modern medicine can alleviate our suffering suggest that traditional norms about the timeliness of disease in human life are being questioned, undermined, and transformed. Baby boomers are not allowed to grow old gracefully. The conflict between disengagement and activity theory represents real changes in the social structure of societies with graying populations, where there are serious social conflicts about the meaning of age and the timeliness of aging. In modern industrial societies, in which there are political conflicts about aging and resources, there is a growing tendency to regard age and aging as socially constructed. Aging can no longer be taken for granted.

NARRATIVE MEDICINE: AIDS AND BIOGRAPHY

Shared narratives of "trouble" (divorce, accident, unemployment, illness, and loss) are important as social supports for the self. Arthur W. Frank (2000) calls these troubles or experiences of alienation "the ride." Illness is a ride on which the patient is involuntarily transported and transformed into a new and strange social environment. Within an intensive-care unit, constant monitoring closes off the normal routines of everyday life, disconnects the everyday but fundamental connections between the body and the self, and converts social reality into a system of alien processes. Frank goes on to claim, however, that "everybody has a story" (2000, 325), the narrative in which hopes, subjectivity, and choices are embedded. These biographical stories make sense of the world of disruptions. But the ride and the story make sense only in a narrative relationship. Thus, Frank says, "I mean by the Ride as a Trope for everything that is not The Story" (323). Patients who survive the ride make an appropriate story, their story, and by sharing the story, they can reenter a normal world of common experiences. Stories are therapeutic devices for reconnecting to social reality.

Individuals who find that their lives are disrupted by sickness and other troubles construct narrative accounts of their lives in an implicit attempt to make sense of the disruptions in their life course. A narrative, like a queue, is a method of introducing a structure into a series of events that might otherwise strike the individual as meaningless, chaotic, and damaging. Narratives may appear to be stories that construct the past in ways that are meaningful, but in fact they are accounts that help individuals see themselves in the future. They locate the troubled individual in a sequence of events that extend into the future, where disruptions may have been successfully resolved. Narratives, in this way, are cultural instruments for sustaining hope and optimism when the present is uncertain and bleak. Narratives can be an important part of therapy. In *At the Will of the Body* (1995), Arthur W. Frank has told the story of his own experiences of cancer. His story, like many cancer tales, is a narrative of survival through pain and anxiety. Telling the story of his cancer is a method of sharing experiences in which other sufferers can see that their experiences are not unique. There is a community of cancer survivors whose narratives give comfort to others because many people survive cancer and those who do not survive can share their stoicism and heroism with others.

Anthropologists and sociologists (Bury 1982; Kleinman 1988; Kleinman and Kleinman 1996) have long recognized the importance of narratives of illness. Narrative theory serves to emphasize the importance of time in human understanding and particularly in the quest for meaning in illness experiences (Ezzy 2000). One unintended consequence of the AIDS crisis has been a deeper appreciation of the importance of narrative in helping people cope with illness by framing a view of the future. People living with HIV/AIDS (PLWHA) confront a dilemma of time (Davies 1997). The AIDS crisis has brought about a particular phase in the development of narrative theory, for three reasons. First, HIV/AIDS has been particularly prevalent in younger groups, and hence many victims have experienced untimely deaths. Second, as demonstrated by Magic Johnson, the basketball hero who eventually spoke openly about his HIV infection, the condition can exist in people who are otherwise supremely fit and athletic. With the development of new drugs, the life expectancy of PLWHA has been extended into an uncertain and difficult future. PLWHA are often young people who have to manage chronic illness over many years, subjecting themselves to strict and demanding medical regimes. Finally, PLWHA are often members of an articulate and educated middle class whose emotional responses to personal crisis have been published as public narrative.

The medical profession has begun to recognize the therapeutic importance of narrative theory. In responding to patients with life-threatening conditions, narrative medicine attempts to encourage or sustain the optimism and trust of patients who may be forced to undertake or accept a prolonged period of medical intervention, much of which will cause them both physical and mental distress. The narrative reconfiguration of time permits the doctor and the patient to cooperate during a treatment that may cause discomfort and allows them to hope that the patient can survive. In the case of such conditions as breast cancer and HIV, there are reasonable medical grounds for looking forward to either recovery or management of the condition. With other conditions, such as oral cancer, the treatment may be severe and the prognosis uncertain or unclear.

In contemporary medicine, there has been a dramatic transformation of attitudes toward providing patients with information about their condition (Salander 2002). In the past, doctors were often secretive about prognoses, allowing patients to live with hope whereas in reality their conditions were terminal. Because doctors are now committed to the disclosure of information, they cannot avoid involvement in the patient's narrative. Although doctors may collude with their patients in the matters of prognosis and the construction of optimism, they also have to convey what is essentially bad news. With difficult forms of cancer, " 'good news' no longer means 'cure,' but remission" (Crossley 2003, 446). Endings are difficult components of a narrative of hope, and hence both patient and doctor may be willing to undertake medical interventions that promise remission in order to delay the introduction of an ending to the narrative.

Endings may be delayed, but they cannot be postponed indefinitely. The precarious nature of the HIV infection may explain why researchers have discovered a variety of narrative structures among PLWHA (Ezzy 2000). With new drug regimes, many HIV sufferers came to assume that they would live into old age and hence constructed "linear restitution narratives" that contained hopeful accounts of returning to a healthy existence, but such narratives are precarious and overly optimistic. By contrast, "linear chaos narratives" exhibit expressions of anger, depression, isolation, and dislocation. They identify the past as healthy and normal and the future as uncertain and bleak. Finally, "polyphonic narratives" express many contradictory positions, combining hope for opportunities for intense living with pessimistic assessments of the longer term.

Endings are important because they remind us that narratives can never be individual or isolated stories. A narrative needs an audience, however small or fragmented. Narratives are typically shared, not only with doctors and nurses but also with friends and relatives. Like all good stories, medical narratives have validity and vitality—in this case because they connect the patient with his or her social network.

It is important to recognize the social and political role of these individual stories as collective narratives. The importance of the collective narrative of AIDS in shaping public attitudes and the research agenda of medicine is a clear example (Hyden 1997). Narratives of suffering restore the victim's social network by setting suffering within a shared culture. The vulnerability of the victim is momentarily relieved as the narrative becomes a shared account of the drama of disease.

The crucial problem with aging and chronic illness is that the isolation of the elderly results in their social detachment and their lack of a social network. Their narratives finally fail for want of an audience.

Narrative theories of the illness experience can be criticized on three grounds. First, by concentrating on the importance of stories of the illness experience for the individual, medical sociology has often neglected an obvious feature of the narratives: they require an audience, and they have a collective force in the dissemination of perspectives on modern illness. Narratives about breast cancer and AIDS, for example, have been crucial in shaping public attitudes toward sufferers and their treatment needs. Second, narrative theory typically neglects the power relationships between the storyteller and the audience. Narratives become authoritative when they have credible sources and influential audiences. Narratives of malaria do not have the same credibility as narratives of AIDS, because they do not have literate, articulate, or influential spokespersons. Finally, it is important to recognize that many narratives—such as narratives of restitution—are important not just in restoring the hope and confidence of patients but in securing patient compliance with demanding medical regimes. It is important to recognize that while doctors and patients might share narratives, the meaningfulness of the ending of the illness experience—such as cure, good health, remission, or death—may not be shared by the participants.

DISRUPTIONS TO SELF AND SOCIETY

If narratives help us understand time in the illness experience, they also provide a window on the social self. In her study of disrupted lives, Gay Becker (1997) follows an established tradition in social anthropology, that of investigating the role of metaphors in traumatic circumstances that produce disruptions of the self. Her research uncovered the important role of metaphors in narratives of disruption and recovery. While her work is grounded in empirical research involving qualitative analysis of victims of various disruptions and disorders, it deductively addresses a theoretical problem: the relationships between the body, metaphors, and identity. Becker's discussion of the consequences of disruption in social life is taken from five separate but interconnected studies—of infertility, midlife crisis, stroke, dependency in old age, and marginality. The notion of "disruption" leads us toward a reflexive uncovering of our vulnerability and the precarious character of our identities.

Sociology and anthropology have demonstrated that identity is fundamentally embodied. Neither our personal identity nor our social identity can be separated from embodiment. It follows that the self is not an enduring or stable fact but evolves with aging and the life course. Hence, radical disruptions to the self occur as a result of traumatic illness, which often destroys our relationships with significant others, transforms our everyday world, and threatens to undermine the comfortable relationship between self, body, and others. In American culture, with its emphasis on youthfulness, activism, and independence, disruptions to everyday life brought on by sickness and aging represent a profound challenge to the sense of self-identity. Because these disruptions can transform the accepted body image, other people may have significant problems in their routine interactions with us—in their responses to the representational ambiguities and the disfigurement of the sick.

Metaphors of illness play an important part in helping people make sense of such unwanted discontinuities. Metaphors not only help us understand disruptions but also have therapeutic qualities. The narratives of disruption are moral accounts of people's lives. Metaphors express the values that make life meaningful and coherent. The idea of a life cycle is itself a metaphor that attempts to express the sense of continuity and accumulation that makes an ordinary life appear satisfactory and meaningful. Narratives of healing are an important part of the healing process. Given the importance of activism and individualism in modern culture, healing narratives are typically structured around the theme of personal responsibility.

It is important not to neglect the role of power relationships in these narratives. In general terms, the hierarchical structure of power in relation to medical knowledge is fundamental to such questions as, What metaphors are available to patients, and how are they legitimized? Are there deviant narratives of illness that subvert medical power? In short, meanings and metaphors are negotiated in medical settings, where resources and knowledge are unequal.

Narratives and metaphors are not universally recognized as beneficial. For example, Susan Sontag, in *Illness as Metaphor* (1978) and *AIDS and Its Metaphors* (1989) complained that metaphors of responsibility could be damaging to the patient. She was in particular critical of the popular notion that people who repress their emotions are more likely to get cancer. In popular psychology and new age movements, being emotional is seen as beneficial. The hidden metaphors here may be related to boiling or percolation: we need to get our emotions out; otherwise, we will boil over and cause ourselves damage. When we are emotional, we often say we are going to burst. The popular notion is that we need to express ourselves to avoid internal damage. Sontag argued that such unhelpful popular metaphors would collapse once an appropriate physical cause of cancer was properly understood. We do not have to accept Sontag's notion of the primacy of physical causes of cancer, but what is clear is that psychosomatic theories that emphasize the importance of expressing emotions are culturally specific. The medical sociologist Colin Samson (1999, 76) points out that for indigenous peoples of the Far North, such as the Inuit, expressing emotions in public is foolhardy and dangerous. If emotional repression were a cause of cancer, we would expect indigenous peoples to have high cancer rates. Paradoxically, increasing cancer rates are associated with their exposure to white society, which promotes emotional expressivity.

The stability of everyday life requires a continuous and reliable conception of the self; hence, disruptions are exceptional interventions within this taken-for-granted normality. We cannot easily or routinely manage everyday interaction without some basic assumptions about continuity and predictability, especially about the stability of identity. The assumptions about stability are constantly challenged, however, especially by the disruption of illness. We are forced to contemplate the permanence of such disruptions. Indeed, perhaps "[c]ontinuity is an illusion. Disruption to life is a constant human experience" (G. Becker 1997, 190). The everyday world involves a constant struggle to sustain the illusions of order and continuity against a backdrop of persistent and ineluctable disorder. If disruptions are in fact continuous disturbances in everyday life, it may be more appropriate to recognize that the temporality of everyday life is one of constant flux.

Disability challenges everyday assumptions because corporeality and embodiment lead directly to questions about the nature of the self. Although disability is socially produced by classification systems and professional labels, it has profound significance for the definition of the self because who we are is necessarily constituted by our embodiment. Since our biographical narratives are carried in our embodiment, disability has to be mediated by its meaning for the self. The day-to-day difficulties of mobility and autonomy are not merely accidental features of the everyday life of the chronically ill, disabled, or elderly; they actually constitute selfhood by transforming the complex relationships between the self, the body image, and the social environment. Disabilities impinge on the everyday capacity of many individuals to make and sustain intimate partnerships; in this respect, the problems of sexual intimacy in old age and chronic illness are not dissimilar (Turner 1995a; Riggs and Turner 1999).

Any account of disruption has to take into account the biography of the individual in terms of whether trauma occurred to a previously regarded whole and healthy person or had its origins in the fetus—that is, whether a person is born with impairment. The temporality of illness emerges through the study of the narrative structure of the self. Disruption is part of the plot of the narration of the self in its social relations, which are themselves temporal. In the sociology of disability, the narrative of Diane DeVries is important for understanding the meaningfulness of disability from the actor's perspective (G. Frank 1984, 1986). DeVries was born without fully developed limbs and therefore had no memory of the "missing limbs." This fact explains why she responded to her official classification as an amputee with amazement. She came, in fact, to think of herself as an image of beauty: an embodiment of the limbless Venus de Milo. Similar experiences of the phenomenology of the body characterize people who are thalidomide victims, because they have no experience of a previous or different type of body. There is an important distinction in studies of disruptions to life involving impairment at birth, accident, and such processes as aging. These three contrasting situations of time and the body have an importance for the sociological understanding of disruptions to the self.

The diseases and discomforts of human beings have their own peculiar temporalities and rhythms—onset, duration, crises, and terminations differ for different diseases and different patients. Some are slow and insidious, others confronting and quick. Oliver Sacks (1976) has given us poetically inspired accounts of the rhythms of chronic sickness and the capacity of drugs to bring about personal awakenings. The availability of new drugs has presented a devastating challenge to chronically ill patients, particularly since they were locked into a time framework that the drugs helped to destroy.

The temporality of disease has different implications for the self. Tourette's syndrome means that the victim is crowded out by an excess of nervous energy that is manifest in a plethora of tics, jerks, grimaces, and noises. In Gilles de la Tourette's clinical notes on this form of "possession," it is observed that no two cases are ever the same, and so the condition has a unique relationship to the self engulfed by the syndrome (Sacks, 1985, 87). The same is true for other impairments and disabilities. We can identify a range of disabilities that are consequences of a traumatic event, such as a traffic or sporting accident. In such cases, the assault on the integrity of the embodied self is massive because there is a clear phenomenological experience of a pretraumatic and posttraumatic personality. The rhythm of disruption is total and abrupt; such accidents require a reconstruction of self and body (Seymour 1998). It is important to distinguish between a sudden traumatic event and a slow and crippling ailment. With rheumatism, the transformations of embodiment are painful but uneven and unpredictable, but the long-term outcome may be physical immobility and social marginality. Finally, some age-related disabilities and impairments cause profound and inevitable loss of mobility, independence, and status (Schieman and Turner 1998; Zola 1988). With aging, however, the loss of mobility and autonomy is an anticipated and possibly normal outcome of the aging process.

Aging, self-identity, and intimacy are linked in a continuous cycle of development (Turner 1995b). The self has to be conceptualized as a process, not an entity. The self is embodied and thus subject to change. What happens to the body is crucial for the integrity and continuity of the self. Gay Becker (1997, 88) argued that "order begins with the body" and "negative representations of old age affect embodied knowledge in late life." Furthermore, monitoring the body for physical impairment is an incessant process in old age. The social gerontologist Mike Hepworth, in his *Stories of Ageing* (2000, 44), records the social importance of mirrors for monitoring the changing self through the aging body. He concludes that "the mirror is not a device for discovering the objective truth about the body but a surface on which we perceive the reflected images of the way we imagine that others see us."

Bodies have a spatial dimension, but they also have temporality. Time is obviously an important factor in the presentation of the self because the "looking-glass image" changes with the life course. This temporality of the body image has an important impact on the notion of self. With the modern emphasis on the beautiful body, the aging process presents an enormous difficulty in terms of maintaining a continuous and valued self. The phenomenological necessity of a continuous self is threatened and undermined by physical aging. With aging, the looking-glass self—that is, the self that is a reflection of how others see us—makes way for the experiential self.

Ontological security is the basis of a person's sense of self. Ontological security involves possessing, on the level of the unconscious and practical consciousness, "answers" to fundamental existential questions of human life (Giddens 1991, 47). Furthermore, a person with a stable sense of self-identity has an experience of biographical continuity, by which he or she is able to manage the contingencies of life. This continuity of the self requires a reflexive endorsement, which is communicated by others (54). As Becker (1997, 12) noted, "[O]ur understanding of ourselves and the world begins with our reliance on the orderly functioning of our bodies," and "we carry our histories with us in the present through our bodies." An illness is a major disruption to biography, and it is existentially necessary to reconstitute a sense of wholeness in order to regain personal continuity (38). Where there is a sudden and unexpected onset of illness, the individual's sense of continuity may disintegrate completely. "Illness necessitates the surrender of the cherished assumption of personal indestructibility" (39).

Following the disruption of everyday life by an acute illness, people experience a period of withdrawal before they can begin to restore a sense of order to their lives; this is true of any form of disruption of the life cycle, such as retirement. The necessary facticity of everyday life means that it cannot be subject to constant or continuous questioning, that is, to systematic reflexivity. Everyday life is not experienced as reflexively present, but it must be taken for granted (Berger and Luckmann 1967, 37). If troublesome occurrences can be explained by commonsense knowledge as something within the parameters of the everyday world, then the disruption is easily integrated into the everyday world (38). The integration of troubles into the everyday world becomes problematic when it is difficult to secure meaningful accounts of abnormal and disruptive events. Untimely disease is by definition an affront to the taken-for-granted nature of the social world within which the self is located. Such dislocations give rise to suffering, the sense of personal alienation, and estrangement from routine circumstances (A. W. Frank 2001).

Conclusion: Time, Careers, and the Corrosion of Character

The shared norms of traditional society, such as the timing of chronic disease in old age, were part of a wider set of assumptions about the life course, careers, and retirement (Turner 1994b). In the early nineteenth century, it was assumed that healthy men could expect to find meaningful employment and have unbroken careers and that women would service the household. In the twentieth century, economic activity was especially important for women. In Britain between 1971 and 1999, women's economic activity increased from 56 to 72 percent. Such high levels of economic participation mask a real change in the nature of the economy and work and obscure a transition from old to new welfare regimes. As a consequence of neoconservative policies in the United States and Britain, the new economic regime is based on monetary stability, fiscal control, and a reduction in government regulation of the economy. This economic strategy did not protect individuals from the uncertainties of the market that dominated welfare strategies between 1930 and 1970, but it helped them participate successfully in the market through education (life-long learning schemes), flexible employment (family-friendly employment strategies), and tax incentives. While the effects of increasing rates of economic activity have been positive, much of the increase in economic participation has required the casualization of the labor force. While the number of men in part-time employment doubled between 1984 and 1999, radical changes in the labor market (job sharing, casualization, flexibility, downsizing, and new management strategies) have disrupted work as a continuous career. For employers, functional and numerical flexibility has broken down rigidities in the workplace but has compromised job security. With the obsolescence of the social relevance of the concept of a career (even among the professional classes), there is an erosion in commitment to the company. Workers can no longer depend on a stable life course or life cycle or a predictable date for retirement.

Downsizing and rightsizing through the displacement of workers create low morale, and low morale leads to poor self-respect. Poor self-respect leads to poor health. These changes in work and career structures constitute what Richard Sennett (1998) has called a "corrosion of character." As the connection between work, identity, and responsibility has been broken by the modern economy, character—a more or less stable public identity—has been changing. Our personal troubles, such as job insecurity and low self-esteem, are consequences of the dynamic nature of the global economy and the transformation of the workplace by technological innovation and structural change.

One consequence is that traditional assumptions about a stable life course organized into definite stages can no longer be sustained. There is little consensus about the characteristics of old age in societies that are changing rapidly. Parsons's presuppositions about the disengagement theory of aging, in which there is an orderly withdrawal from society, are not relevant to a society in which the retirement age is flexible. And people have many occupations rather than careers. Modern technology also holds out the promise of the management of aging through biological and technological intervention. This vision of the technological modification of aging points to a utopian world in which aging is no barrier to self-development, experimentation, or adventure. According to other social analysts, a wealthy minority will achieve this utopian dream, but the majority of aging people in modern societies with an emphasis on youthfulness and activism will experience isolation, marginality, and alienation. These contrasting images of aging, as either passive or active, are reflections of uncertain and divided cultures that produce many unresolved narratives of aging. In such societies, the social consensus on the timeliness of disease and sickness or on the structure of the life course of the individual is tenuous and fragmented. Narratives of aging are contested because there is little agreement about the normal life course.

Chapter Five
RESHAPING HEALTH AND ILLNESS

INTRODUCTION: AGING, DISABILITY, AND DEATH

THE GRAYING OF THE POPULATIONS of Western societies is changing the nature of disease, especially by increasing disability and chronic illness. Aging populations also transform the issues that confront modern medicine and health-care systems because an aging population places a significant financial burden on health-care costs, especially when retirement is compulsory. The germ theory and the biomedical model that were prominent features of the success of scientific medicine in the nineteenth and early twentieth century have less relevance to the understanding and treatment of the chronic conditions of old age. The health problems associated with an aging population—diabetes, heart disease, dementia, impairment, and disability—require different interventions and social policies, ones that address dependency, isolation, and chronicity. My primary interest is the social consequences of impairment and disability with aging, but it is also important to look at how these changes to society are experienced by the individual and how they affect self-conceptions as a consequence of impairments to embodiment.

In recent years, the remarkable development of critical gerontology has led to the questioning of many conventional assumptions about the classification of age and aging. Of particular importance in this field are Stephen Katz's *Disciplining Old Age* (1996) and Bryan S. Green's *Gerontology and the Construction of Old Age* (1993). These works reflect the general importance of Foucault in the study of the science of aging in the new medical sociology. Both Katz and Green address the question, how did older people become classified as "the elderly," and what was the role of scientific gerontology in bringing about the governance of the elderly? Although these perspectives are useful in questioning the classificatory systems of gerontology, they do not offer any insight into the experience of aging—namely, into the problems of elderly embodiment.

Foucauldian studies of aging explore how the elderly became a special subject of science studied from the point of view of medicine and how their characteristic complaints became the concern of a special set of disciplines that are orchestrated by gerontology. Older people have become a matter of increasing economic and political interest. Before the Industrial Revolution, people older than sixty-five constituted less than 3 percent of the population. By 2030 in the developed world, one-quarter of the population will be older than sixty-five. At present, the "dependency ratio" is three workers to one retiree. By 2030 in Germany and Italy, it will be one to one. In the 1960s, the worldwide fertility rate (average number of lifetime births per woman) was five. Today it is less than three, and the population-replacement rate is two live births per woman. A shrinking workforce in an aging world is economically and militarily problematic, and thus in the view of economic analysts "graying means paying." In industrialized societies, it is alleged that paying for "promised benefits" to pensioners in this century will involve an increase in the total tax burden by as much as 40 percent. It is hardly surprising that growing old has increasingly become a target of medical interest.

In 1481, the word *senectitude* meant "old age," and by 1695 *senescence* referred to the process of growing old. By 1791, *senility* was a state of being old, and in 1848 *senile* meant "weak." At the end of the nineteenth century, old age had been converted into a pathological state (Katz 1996). The changing meanings of *senility* indicate that the elderly have become a burden from the point of view of economic efficiency. In the United States before 1900, 67 percent of men over age sixty-five were still employed. This figure was 31 percent in 1951, 25 percent in 1961, 19 percent in 1971, and 16 percent in 1976. The elderly are being excluded from employment through compulsory and historically fixed retirement regulations. The social and political response to aging has been to regulate the elderly through a new set of disciplines and practices that fall under the rubric of scientific gerontology.

With the graying of society, there has been a significant increase in chronic illness, disability, and dependence. Of course, how we measure or quantify impairment is itself a problematic issue that makes the formulation of social policies for the elderly difficult (Fujiura and Rutkowski-Kmitta 2001). The disability rate per capita in the developed world is higher than that in the less developed societies of the third world, partly as a consequence of the methods of data collection and partly because the rapid aging of Western societies inevitably produces more disabled people. Regardless of the problems of defining and collecting data on aging, disability and impairment begin to increase in the over-fifty age group, with a particularly steep increase after sixty years of age. Causes of disability and impairment are complex, however, and should be distinguished. The principal causes of disability are arthritis and problems of the circulatory system, while the main causes of impairment are disease, illness, congenital abnormalities, and injury. There is also a new range of causes of disability arising from HIV infections and hepatitis. Finally, it is important to grasp the importance of disability as a global problem with a severe impact on economic performance. It is estimated that there are between 235 million and 549 million disabled people in the world (Albrecht and Verbrugge 2000).

The transformation of the demographic structure of society has increased awareness of the isolation and loneliness of older people and the problems of dying and bereavement in modern society, where family and kinship structures fail to provide adequate support for the elderly. Alongside a new wave of research on the elderly, there has been an intellectually exciting development of disability studies, in which sociological insight has been influenced by the consequences of the growth of a politics of disability. Whereas mainstream sociology conveniently neglected disability and impairment, recent critical work in this field has raised questions that are important for a general understanding of social movements and politics (Albrecht, Seelman, and Bury 2001). When the family disintegrates as a support system, the problems of aging and disability are magnified, and the voluntary sector is expected to take a larger share of the burden of dependency (Brown, Kenny, and Turner 2000). As a consequence, disability and impairment become important dimensions of social citizenship and human rights in contemporary societies (Barnes, Mercer, and Shakespeare 1999).

The graying of the population has also produced an interest in the sociology of death and dying. We have already seen that symbolic interactionism and grounded theory made important contributions to the study of dying in the late 1960s (Glaser and Strauss 1965, 1968b; Sudnow 1967). These academic developments are illustrated by the growth of new journals such as *Mortality* (from 1996), a critical textbook on palliative medicine (Doyle, Hanks, and MacDonald 1998), and the emergence of a new sociological field, the sociology of death and dying (Mulkay and Ernst 1991). The rise of "death studies" and the secular proliferation of occupational groups related to death and dying are witnesses to an erosion of traditional social structures and the growing specialization of the treatment of the dying (Hallam, Hockey, and Howarth 1999).

THE DISABILITY MOVEMENT

Disability has been neglected until recently within both mainstream sociology (Ingstad and Whyte 1995) and the humanities (D. T. Mitchell and Snyder 1997). Nor has the cultural meaning of the body and disability received the attention it deserves (Thomas 2002). Apart from influential work by Erving Goffman (1964) and the medical sociologist Irving Zola (1982, 1988), sociology has contributed surprisingly little to the study of disability in terms of systematic theory and research. In the study of mental health and social deviance, symbolic interactionism produced an influential literature, which gave rise to radical criticism of taken-for-granted notions of normality and questioned the conventional distinctions between norm, normal, and deviance (S. J. Williams 1987). Grounded theory has addressed important issues in the analysis of chronic illness (Strauss and Glaser 1975).

The sociological understanding of disability was initially influenced by research on labeling, stigma, and deviance. While conventional criminology accepted a narrow legal definition of crime and deviance, deviancy studies argued that deviance is in the eye of the beholder, and sociological research consequently concentrated on the processes of deviance and deviancy amplification. The sociology of disability was initially somewhat submerged in studies of stigma and stigmatization (Goffman 1964). Symbolic interactionism developed an array of useful concepts around the idea of "discredited" and "discreditable" identities and studied the management of interaction between "normals" and the chronically sick and disabled (F. Davis 1963). In a similar fashion, disability in medical sociology has not been a major research interest. Studies of disability have typically appeared in research on aging, where it is represented under the heading of "dependency" (Hocking and James 1993). In this context, disability became associated with negative "images of aging" (Featherstone and Wernick 1995).

This situation of relative scientific neglect changed in the 1980s and 1990s, however, with the growth of the disability movement and the political quest for social rights. The social theory of Peter Berger and Thomas Luckmann (1966) on "the social construction of reality" facilitated the development of the disability movement in that their analysis of the social organization of knowledge provided a basis for the social model of disability. Their social theory promoted the views that disability is socially constructed and that disability, rather than being a self-evident physical dysfunction, is the product of social processes. This sociological approach was important in recasting disability as a loss of civil rights rather than simply a taken-for-granted impairment (Nagi 1976).

As a result, there is greater public awareness of the notion that the prejudicial assumptions of the media and the deployment of a "disabling language" reinforce negative stereotypes (Auslander and Gold 1999). It is now recognized that there is an ideology of ableism that has exclusionary social functions. As a result, writers like Wendy Seymour (1989, 1998) have more systematically analyzed the negative consequences of the medicalization of patients and the use of the biomedical model in rehabilitation. This emphasis on ability as an assumption of the dominant culture may be particularly true of American society, in which the twentieth-century "youth complex" gave a salient position to individualism, achievement, and success (Parsons 1999b). Youthfulness became the principal criterion for aesthetic judgments of the body. As a result, ableism underpins more general values about the cultural importance of sports, athleticism, and masculinity; the notion of physical dexterity becomes an index of more general distinction. In contemporary consumer societies, the youthful and powerful body has increasingly become a sign of social worth; the body has become a principal theme in the notion of the self as a project. Against a background of relative neglect, there has been an emerging critical literature on disability that has had an effect on the social sciences, where ideas of disability, handicap, and impairment are now thoroughly contested (Barnes, Mercer, and Shakespeare 1999). These intellectual changes were anticipated by Zola's critical lecture on "bringing bodies back in" (1991). In this chapter, I attempt to show that both politically and analytically there is a growing appreciation of the body and embodiment in modern sociology and that the sociology of the body can make important contributions to the study of impairment and disability (Thomas 2002).

This chapter has three aims. The first is to develop a sociology of the body that combines an appreciation of the phenomenology of the body in the everyday world and an awareness that the body is constructed as an object of professional concern. To this end, I examine both the subjectivity of the "lived body" (Toombs 1995; Zola 1991) and the external social and political structures that regulate, produce, and govern bodies and populations in the Foucauldian tradition (Burchell, Gordon, and Miller 1991). This argument depends on a distinction between the notions of embodiment and the government of the body. The term *embodiment* attempts to describe the phenomenological subjectivity of the lived body in the life world, whereas *governmentality* describes the production of the body as an object of professional knowledge and practice. The second aim is to examine vulnerability and contingency in relation to the embodied self in order to disrupt further the idea of "natural" disability. Finally, I consider how a sociology of the body can provide an analysis of human and social rights that is grounded in the social ontology of human beings as both frail and vulnerable. These three points serve the same critical purpose: to provide an inquiry into the Cartesian dualism of mind and body in order to situate the sociology of the body at the center of disability debates.

In exploring the relevance of sociology to an understanding

of disability, we should briefly rehearse two versions of the sociology of the body in contemporary social thought that have been explored in earlier chapters. The first is the Foucauldian debate about the social production of the human body, which leads to an analysis of how disability is socially constructed. Such an approach is radical in the sense that it treats the rehabilitation process, for example, as normalization, demonstrating how the "disabled body" is discursively produced, governed, and regulated. The management of disability is a form of governmentality (Rose 1989, 5), a development of microsystems of social regulation that exercise normative control over individuals and populations. In this sense, rehabilitation is a form of governmentality that orchestrates various medical and welfare practices that aim to create the rehabilitated person. The second version of the sociology of the body we need to consider if we are to understand the problems of disability in everyday life comprehensively is a phenomenology of the impaired body.

Disability and Social Construction

In sociology, there has been a deep division between social constructionism and phenomenology. Although these traditions are typically regarded as irreconcilable, in this chapter, for an analysis of disability, I seek a theoretical rapprochement between Foucault's poststructuralism and Maurice Merleau-Ponty's phenomenology (Turner 1992, 1995a, 1997b, 1996). There are different levels to the study of disability—namely, individuals' experience of disability, the social organization of disability in terms of sociocultural categories, the macro, or societal, level of welfare provision, and the politics of disability

(Barnes, Mercer, and Shakespeare 1999, 35). Foucault's idea of normalization is useful in understanding how medical interventions standardize human experience, but a phenomenology of the body provides a basis for a better appreciation of the actual experiences and subjectivity of embodiment. This chapter is consistent with the position taken by Susan Reynolds Whyte (1995, 276), who has criticized Foucault and Henri-Jacques Stiker as frameworks for analysis of individuals' experiences of misfortune, disease, and disability because "[d]iscourse analysis does not leave much room for their subjectivity and agency." Whyte argues that the ethnographic tradition of anthropology has therefore much to offer the exploration of the subjective experiences of the everyday world, an issue about which discourse analysis is silent.

"Disability" is, in terms of the sociology of knowledge, not unlike "gender" in that its very existence has been questioned by the politics of constructionism. The Union of the Physically Impaired Against Segregation (UPIAS) defines disability in terms of citizenship, as a loss of social and political opportunities. This social model of disability is highly appropriate for advocacy purposes because it directs attention to inadequate social provision. In this perspective, society creates disability out of people with impairments (Bickenbach 1993).

The disability movement has been based on the creation of a "social model" of disability, which is a direct challenge to the medical model. A medical model regards both disease and sickness as medical conditions that are produced by a specific entity (such as a bacterium) and assumes that the role of medical intervention is to control the symptoms of a disease and, where possible, remove the causes of disease and suffering. It does not attend to the subjective worldview of patients as constitutive of the condition and does not readily recognize the role of politics and culture in shaping human illness (Turner 1995b, 1998a). By "focusing on the ways in which disability is socially produced, the social model has succeeded in shifting debate about disability from agendas dominated by biomedicine to discourses about politics and citizenship" (Hughes and Paterson 1997, 325). This displacement is made possible, however, by an unsatisfactory division between the concepts of impairment and disability. By defining disability as a social and political condition of exclusion and viewing impairment as a medical category describing an absent or defective limb, organism, or mechanism of the body, the social construction of the disabled body confines impairment to a medical framework. While a constructionist interpretation of the body liberates disability, the medical model still dominates the field of impairment.

Postmodern and poststructuralist theories that regard the body as a text or script from which we can read the significance of modern society have effectively banished the palpable, living body from analysis, because postmodern perspectives preclude the possibility of an "ethnography of physicality" (Shakespeare and Watson 1995, 16) that would be highly valuable to the disability movement. Postmodern ethnographic methodology has been important in demonstrating that social science has to listen to the many voices that emerge from fieldwork, but the cultural relativism of anthropological research often prohibits the development of an active politics of intervention (Cowan, Dembour, and Wilson 2001). Because postmodernism is attentive to the contested interpretations of social life, postmodern studies of the human body have rejected methodological realism in favor of deconstructing representations of the human body. The consequence has been the transformation of the living body into a cultural system and the loss of the physical dimension of impairment and embodiment (S. J. Williams 1999).

Ethnographic research provides an important insight into the unique experience of impairment and its individual consequences. Wendy Seymour's moving account of the experience and treatment of spinal cord injury provides an illustration of an ethnographic approach to the physicality of the impaired body that transcends the artificial separation of the objective and subjective body. *Remaking the Body* (1998) and *Bodily Alterations* (1989) are studies of trauma that open up new directions in the study of disability. Employing qualitative data from interviews, Seymour examined the social construction of the body in a literal sense: the way bodies are remade following trauma from accident or disease. This posttraumatic rebuilding of the body also involves a "second chance" at refashioning the self (Giddens 1991). The therapeutic remaking of the body—through training, exercise, and discipline—is not merely a discursive process, because it involves the reconstruction of the lived, sensual body. This remaking of the body also takes place within the professional "gaze" of rehabilitation, which holds out the misleading promise of normalization and the production of a socially "normal" body—young, athletic, and sexual. It is not enough to return to society via rehabilitation; the rehabilitated body has to be discursively normal. Seymour's ethnographic study showed how, through endless medical and psychological encounters in the rehabilitation process, individuals are coached, coaxed, and often cajoled to pick up the vestiges of normal and routine social roles in a narrative of restitution.

IMPAIRMENT AND DISABILITY

One solution to conceptual difficulties with the medical and social models of disability has been to synthesize those processes into a biopsychosocial model. Such a model was incorporated into the International Classification of Impairments, Disabilities, and Handicaps (ICIDH) proposals of WHO in 1997, in which every dimension of disablement is analyzed in terms of an interaction between the individual and his or her social and physical environment. We can also view this model as a sequential development from impairment to disability. There is, first, the onset of impairments that involve anatomical or structural abnormalities of organs, parts of the body, or whole bodies. These produce functional limitations that can be both physical and mental. Finally, there is disability, which refers to difficulties in performing social roles (Jette 1999). As a result of this development, there are three disablement pathways, namely, impairments, activities, and participation.

The model assumes that different types of intervention are appropriate at different levels. While medical intervention may be appropriate in relation to the specific features of impairment, sociopolitical action is appropriate at the level of the disability. Disability is hence a loss of the full benefits of citizenship and requires political and social change to contain the negative effects of impairment. Although movement activists have criticized the model because it labels individuals in terms of an official and professional system of classification, others have claimed that it transcends the limitations of both the social and the medical models and holds out the promise of a more universalistic approach (Bickenbach et al. 1999). Although the idea of a synthesis is attractive, to argue that the biological should not be dismissed is quite separate from an account of human embodiment. From the perspective of sociology, "the body" is not in some elementary framework "the biological." The point of the sociology of embodiment is to go beyond a Cartesian medical framework in which mind-body dualism is replaced; there is little advantage in substituting a psychology-biology dualism for the traditional mind-body dualism.

Contemporary studies of the phenomenology of impairment and disability further question the legacy of mind-body dualism. The sociology of disability demonstrates the limitations of a simple mind-body dualism and takes us into a discussion of the embodied self and the disruptions of everyday life. The nature of corporeality and embodiment leads directly to the question of the self and the social actor (Charmaz 1994; Deegan 1978; Oberg 1996). Disability, while socially produced by systems of classification and professional labels, also has profound significance for the self because our identity is necessarily constituted by our embodiment. Since our biographical narratives are embodied, disability is an existential challenge in terms of its contested meaning for the self. The problems of mobility and autonomy are fundamental to the life world of the disabled. Disability shapes selfhood by transforming the relationships between the self, body image, and social world. These disabilities impinge on the practical capacity of individuals to make intimate partnerships.

Disability and the Politics of the Body

This issue of the body as distinct from embodiment of the social actor also has to be cast in a historical context. Sociologists are not only concerned with the phenomenology of the embodied self; they must also recognize that the relationship between body and society differs with time and place and therefore the debate about the relationship between selfhood and disability shifts. In contemporary Western societies, the context is an individualistic and hedonistic culture with an emphasis on youth, youthfulness, and activity. For example, critical gerontology emphasizes activity and engagement as opposed to the idea that successful aging requires disengagement (Phillipson 1998, 15–16). This emphasis on the youthful, active, slim body is connected to the importance of reflexivity as a component of modernity. Recent writing has associated the emergence of the debate about the body with the growing importance of the postmodern, or reflexive, self. For example, Anthony Synnott (1993, 1) has asserted that "the body is also, and primarily, the self. We are all embodied." Following sociological approaches to contemporary forms of intimacy (Giddens 1991, 1992), Chris Shilling argued (1993, 1) that the project of the self in modern society is in fact the project of the body: "there is a tendency for the body to become increasingly central to the modern person's sense of self-identity."

Medical technology has made possible the construction of the human body as a personal project through cosmetic surgery, organ transplants, prosthetics, and transsexual surgery. In addition, there is the panoply of dieting regimes, health farms, sports science, and nutritional science that concentrates on the development of the aesthetic, thin body. Both Synnott and Shilling have noted that modern sensibility and subjectivity are focused on the physical body as a representation of the self, such that the body in contemporary society is a mirror of one's personality. There has been a profound process of secularization whereby diet is transformed from a discipline of the body that constrained the Christian soul into a secular mechanism for the expression of sexuality; in turn, our sexuality is a framework of modern selfhood (Turner 1996). Whereas traditional forms of diet subordinated the passions in the interests of the salvation of the soul, in the contemporary consumer society, diet assumes an entirely different meaning and importance, as an elaboration or amplification of sexuality. We want to be thin in order to be sexual. The project of the self is intimately bound up with these historical transformations of the nature of the body, its role in culture, and its location in the public sphere. Although sociologists have invested much effort in understanding cosmetic surgery as a technique for refashioning the self through body transformations, there is, as we have noted in the work of Seymour, an important system of rehabilitation in contemporary medicine and social work that contributes to rebuilding the self and normalizing the body. Self-help groups and popular health literature play an important part in promoting the idea that looking good is the first step toward not just feeling good but being good. Given this emphasis on the beautiful body in the commercial culture of contemporary capitalism, there is an "aestheticisation of everyday life" that puts considerable social pressure on conformity within these health norms (Radley 1999). Both old bodies and impaired bodies need rehabilitation in order to conform to the values of youthfulness, beauty, and athleticism. In contemporary America, even short-ness of stature, especially among men, is a cause of anxiety and, potentially, a medical condition. The election of small men to such political offices as the presidency is problematic; the size of the presidential role requires the presence of a large and handsome American body. Bill Clinton perfectly embodied the ideal of a healthy, charismatic leader, whereas an old and infirm political leader indicates a tired and ailing government. The word *ailment* is derived from the Old English *egl(i)an*, indicat-ing "troublesome" (*egle*) and, in its Gothic form, "disgraceful" (*agls*); an ailing body is seen to be without grace (charisma).

Impairment can assume many forms. While the sociology of deafness is an underdeveloped area of research (Higgins 1980), deafness provides an important example of the social and polit-ical issues that surround impairment. The struggle over the so-cial rights of deaf people illustrates the processes of exclusion that frequently attend impairment. The contemporary history of educational responses to signed languages has been sympa-thetically captured in Oliver Sacks's *Seeing Voices* (1989), which shows how the traditional response to deafness, especially to the prelingual deaf, was to regard it as a calamity. Those who were unable to acquire speech were automatically labeled "dumb" or "mute." Before the late eighteenth century, there was little prospect that the deaf could acquire any education, and hence they were effectively segregated from society. Med-ical interest in the diseases of the ear began in France in the seventeenth century, and James Hinton in London and Rudolf Schwartze in Halle, Germany, developed the mastoidectomy in the early nineteenth century, but the important advances were educational rather than medical. In 1755, Abbé Charles-

Michel de l'Epée founded a school in France to teach signed language, whereby students could write down what was communicated to them through a signing interpreter. L'Epée's interest in signed language was a product of Enlightenment debates about the origin of language and whether a universal language had existed prior to the differentiation of modern languages. He believed that what he called the "mimicry" of the deaf was the root of such a foundational language. By the time of his death, in 1789, he had established twenty-one schools for the deaf in Europe, and in 1791 the National Institution of Deaf-Mutes was established in Paris.

L'Epée's pedagogy had a dramatic impact on social attitudes toward the deaf. The eighteenth-century philosopher Étienne Condillac, who explored the origin of language and the creation of symbols, regarded the deaf as "sentient statues," incapable of thought. On seeing l'Epée's pupils, he became a convert to the beneficial effects of education and the use of signed language. In the United States, influenced by l'Epée's disciples, Thomas Hopkins Gallaudet and Laurent Clerc established the American Asylum for the Deaf and Dumb in Hartford, Connecticut, in 1817. The French sign system, which was imported by Clerc, was rapidly amalgamated with indigenous signing conventions, and American Sign Language (ASL) evolved under the influence of deaf people from Martha's Vineyard, Massachusetts, who came to Hartford during its early years. In 1864, Congress passed a law recognizing the Columbia Institution for the Deaf and the Dumb and the Blind in Washington, D.C., as a national deaf-mute college, and by 1869 about 41 percent of teachers of the deaf in the United States were themselves deaf.

These principles of educational reform for the deaf were continued in America until 1870, when there was a rapid and profound reversal of philosophy. The success of ASL meant that deaf people were able to acquire education, but it also reinforced the social solidarity of the deaf as a distinctive community with its own language, educational system, and values. Signed language recognized the difference of the deaf and celebrated their social distinctiveness. Toward the end of the nineteenth century, there was a new emphasis on assimilation and conformity, and cultural differences were regarded as divisive and unwanted. The assimilationist mood was expressed through an emphasis on speech rather than signed language, and "oralist" educators set up "progressive" educational institutions that ignored signing and imposed a curriculum that required speech. The Clarke School for the Deaf in Northampton, Massachusetts, was opened in 1867 to teach speech, and at the International Congress of Educators of the Deaf in Milan, Italy, in 1880, where deaf teachers were excluded from a vote, the use of signed language was officially proscribed.

The effects of this philosophy were dramatic. Whereas almost half of all teachers of the deaf in the United States were deaf in 1850, the proportion declined to one-quarter in 1900 and to 12 percent in 1960. The costs of speech education are prohibitive. According to Sacks (1989, 30), deaf people show no "native disposition whatever to speak," and speaking is an ability that must be laboriously taught to them. By contrast, they have an immediate propensity to sign and achieve considerable fluency by the age of fifteen months. The underlying problem is that those outside the deaf community do not regard signed language as a "proper language" and hence contend that it requires the supplement of speech or, indeed, the replacement of signed language by speech. As a result of the impact of the civil rights movement and the political organization of the deaf themselves, social attitudes began to change in the 1970s. The social and political problem is that while deafness is an impairment of hearing, it has been transformed into a disability, whereby social rights and status have been denied. There is a Deaf culture and a Deaf community, whose members include people with a congenital hearing impairment and hearing people who have grown up in the ASL community because they are children of deaf people. This community is held together culturally by a separate and distinctive language and by the experiences of exclusion and stigmatization (L. J. Davis 1996). In this case study of deafness, we can detect an important illustration of the intersection of bodily impairment, the historical stigma of being a "deaf-mute," and the mobilization of a community to achieve social citizenship.

BODY AND TIME

Although embodiment is a social project routinely accomplished with comfort or ease, it also has its own specificity. My embodiment is uniquely accomplished within wholly routine and predictable contexts. We can express this paradox of particularity and uniformity in terms of the relationship between sociology and ontology in Martin Heidegger's *Question of Being* (1958). On the social or horizontal plane, an individual is routinely defined by a series of social roles that specify a standardized position in society. There is also an ontological plane, which forms a vertical axis that is defined by the finite and unique embodiment of a person. The horizontal social plane represents the precarious world of the social system. The vertical plane is the life world within which human beings are embodied and vulnerable. In this sense, we might argue that sociological (horizontal) analysis seeks to understand the contingent and arbitrary characteristics of social being while the philosophical (vertical) analysis attempts to grasp the existential limitations of being. This formulation can be adopted as a further perspective on Foucault's notion of the arbitrariness of institutions. The horizontal plane of social relations is both arbitrary and precarious. The institutions of disability and rehabilitation have been radically transformed in the late twentieth century, and the traditional systems of rehabilitation no longer hold sway. On the vertical plane of human existence, however, there are certain necessities concerned with aging, disability, and dependency. This way of formulating the relationship between society and individual is useful in reminding us that with aging, the majority of the population will experience physical and mental impairment, limitations, and disabilities. The concept of universal vulnerability is useful because it underscores the fact that disability is not a peculiar circumstance of an unfortunate minority. Vulnerability is a condition in which we all share, and we all confront the possibility of physical impairment and disability.

In many respects, the notion of disruption by disease captures the relationship between these vertical and horizontal dimensions. The disruptions we experience with disease uncover our vulnerability and open opportunities for self-reflection. These disruptions of our illness experiences expose our personal vulnerability and further illustrate the inadequacies of the Cartesian legacy of the mind-body dichotomy. Both sociology and anthropology have demonstrated that identity is fundamentally embodied. I cannot have a more or less stable identity unless I can be recognized in social settings, and recognition depends in part on a more or less continuous embodiment. DNA testing has meant that traditional forms of recognition of public identities by police lineups and fingerprinting are slowly becoming obsolete, but my recognition in everyday life still rests on the presentation of an embodied self. Hence my identity cannot be easily separated from my embodiment.

It follows that self is not an enduring or stable fact but changes with aging, the life course, and the disruptions of illness and injury. Hence, radical disruptions to the self occur as a result of traumatic illness, accident, or injury. The disruptions of illness often shatter our relationships with significant others, force us out of employment, reorganize our life world, and threaten to destroy the comfortable relationship between self, body, and others. In modern societies, where there is an emphasis on activism and autonomy, disruptions to everyday life from accident, chronic illness, and aging represent a profound challenge to self-identity. Talcott Parsons's sick role (1951) defined sickness in terms of inactivity; to be sick was essentially not to be at work. In a society that values activism, chronic illness and impairment are in this sense deviant (A. W. Frank 1991b; Gerhardt 1987). In America and Britain, where social rights are based on previous contributions in terms of work, military service, or parenting, disability is stigmatized because it is associated with unemployment (Albrecht 1992). In Sweden and Denmark, the social democratic tradition of welfare does not regard welfare rights as a repayment of contributions made through work and taxation but argues that welfare entitlements exist to satisfy the needs of citizens. As a result, the fact that many disabled people cannot work does not mean that they are automatically stigmatized.

DISABILITY AND RIGHTS

There is pressure within the social sciences, as in medicine, to "normalize" the body, whereby a body with impairment is an unusual or abnormal body in need of compassion (Rock 2000). The development of the disability-adjusted life year (DALY) by the World Bank and WHO was intended to provide an objective basis for the cost-effective analysis of health programs, but it has had the effect of promoting a utilitarian norm of the universal human body. Disability activists emphasize the human rights aspect of disability and argue that it is a normal condition in all human populations. In the search for perfect health and the "normal" body, we should not exclude disability and impairment by treating them as pathologies. The disability movement has been critical of the "experience of illness" approach because it detracts from what is regarded as the real issue—the lack of social rights. Any account of disability should therefore attempt to frame the problem in the context of social and human rights.

Both impairment and aging are important illustrations of our vulnerability (Turner 2000c, 2001a). While age as a system of social classification and aging as a social process are culturally defined, the physical consequences of the aging process are inevitable. The process is individually variable, but our immune systems tend to decline with age, and our exposure to physical impairments increases as we grow older. The great majority of people will experience some form of disability in old age, and there is a definite experience of a loss of mastery after age sixty (Mirowsky 1995). Human beings as embodied creatures are subject to illness, disease, aging, and mental decay through dementia, Alzheimer's disease, Parkinson's disease, and so forth. We can derive the need for protective human rights from this Hobbesian notion that human beings are biologically frail, socially vulnerable, and politically precarious (Turner 1997a). Human beings manage their "ontological security" (Giddens 1991, 44) through the development of everyday routines. These routines are prone to fail because our social and political world is precarious. Daily routines and norms are constantly and unpredictably disrupted because our embodiment means that we are exposed to physical risks. We are also routinely disappointed by everyday life because our normative expectations are constantly challenged by these failures and shortcomings. Historically, the narratives of religion and medicine have provided us with compensating theodicies to support the everyday-world explanations that make our misfortunes appear meaningful and hence acceptable (Berger 1969). The sinfulness of human beings provided, in traditional Christianity, an explanation of the misfortunes of illness.

In addition to being biologically frail, we are vulnerable at a social level. The aging process provides a clear illustration of the precariousness of social arrangements. As we age in chronological and biological terms, we are increasingly exposed to our vulnerability because, particularly in modern society, old age is a period of growing isolation and loneliness. We cannot easily provide for our own wants and needs, and we become dependent on family and kinship networks. With growing longevity in societies where traditional family systems have broken down, the elderly become increasingly dependent and excluded. Biological frailty and social vulnerability tend to reinforce the problems of marginality and isolation that the sick, disabled, and elderly experience. Their social marginality often results in abuse and domestic violence. Eric Klinenberg, in *Heat Wave* (2002), has shown how elderly and isolated men were particularly exposed to the health hazards of extreme summer temperatures in Chicago.

Social institutions are precarious. Institutions, which are rationally designed to serve specific purposes, may evolve in ways that contradict their original charters. Social life is essentially contingent and risky; individuals, even when they come together in concerted action, cannot necessarily protect themselves from the vagaries of social reality. We are precarious at the societal level because we cannot effectively control macropolicy decisions on such issues as compulsory retirement, mandatory retirement contributions, inheritance taxation, health coverage, and so forth. Poverty, or lack of social resources, is an important aspect of social precariousness, and precariousness means social disruption or low social capital. In the United States, one objective measure of this weakness of the social fabric is the fact that approximately 40 million Americans have no medical insurance coverage. They are seriously exposed to the whimsical character of illness episodes.

Following the American pragmatist philosopher Richard Rorty (1998), a theory of human rights can be derived from certain aspects of feminist theory, from a critical view of the limitations of utilitarianism, and from an understanding of the proper role of sentiment and emotion in human character. Insofar as the strong protect the weak, it is because there is a recognition of likeness that produces the conditions for affective attachment and sentiment. People want their rights to be recognized because they see in the plight of other human beings their own potential or actual unhappiness and misery (Turner 1997a, 1998b). Because individual aging is an inevitable biological process, we can in principle anticipate our own dependence, vulnerability, and frailty. While the notion of sympathy has received bad press in modern societies, it is crucial in deciding to whom our moral concern might be directed. Sympathy derives from the fundamental experiences of dependency and reciprocity in everyday life, particularly from the relationship between mother and child.

If this argument is to prevail, we need to elaborate the notion of human frailty by developing a distinction between pain and suffering. Human beings can suffer without an experience of pain, and conversely they can have an experience of pain without suffering. Suffering is essentially a situation in which the self is threatened or destroyed by events over which we may have little control. We can suffer the loss of a loved one without physical pain, whereas a toothache may give us extreme physical pain without a sense of suffering or humiliation. While suffering is variable, pain might be regarded as universal. Suffering depends on how the self is defined culturally, whereas the sudden pain of a toothache is relatively unmediated by cultural assumptions (Kleinmann, Das, and Lock 1997).

There is an additional claim that can be made: while pleasures are variable, human misery is universal. Although we find it difficult to agree on a definition of happiness, there is little disagreement as to the nature of human suffering (B. Moore

1970). This argument is closely related to a position adopted by Richard Rorty in *Contingency, Irony, and Solidarity* (1989, 88), in which he argues that "the idea that we have an overriding obligation to diminish cruelty, to make human beings equal in respect of their liability to suffering, seems to take for granted that there is something within human beings which deserves respect and protection quite independently of the language they speak. It suggests that a non-linguistic ability, the ability to feel pain, is what is important, and the differences in the vocabulary are much less important."

Vulnerability is a universal condition of the human species because pain is a fundamental experience of all organic life. Such an argument about our vulnerable condition runs counter to the conventional anthropological view of cultural relativism (Ingstad and Whyte 1995; Stiker 1982). Anthropology argues that cultures are variable and there could be no consensus about vulnerability across cultures. It is possible to defend the idea of vulnerability against anthropological relativism by employing the distinction between pain and suffering. The latter is culturally variable because cultures have different definitions of suffering as a loss of respect, but there is a neurological foundation to pain that is not entirely subject to cultural context. It is unlikely that we will discover a society in which tooth decay is not experienced as a painful event (Turner and Rojek 2001). Zola (1989) has defended moral universalism against cultural relativism with respect to disability and impairment. He was acutely aware of the paradox, or "dilemma of difference" (Goffman 1964): political demands to end various forms of discrimination require a social analyst to identify those who are experiencing discrimination. This identification of a minority requires a special focus on the difference, but to ignore the difference delays the development of positive policies against discrimination. Against a "special needs approach," Zola argued (1989, 406) that in the long term we need to support universal policies that recognize that the entire population is in some sense "at risk" in terms of chronic illness and disability. He took this universalistic stance, because "[o]nly when we acknowledge the near universality of disability and that its dimensions (including the biomedical) are part of the social process by which the meanings of disability are negotiated will it be possible fully to appreciate how general public policy can affect this issue."

The aging of the populations of Western society, the growing prevalence of chronicity, and the globalization of health risks are important demographic and sociological aspects of Zola's understanding of the universality of disability. For the social sciences, the challenge of Zola's view of embodiment must remain a permanent feature of both disability studies and policy formation: only by "bringing bodies back in" can an adequate sociology of disability finally be created.

Chapter Six
GENDER, SEXUALITY, AND THE BODY

INTRODUCTION: IDENTITY AND THE DISCOURSE OF SEXUALITY

THE NEW MEDICAL SOCIOLOGY addresses many of the key issues of modern social structure and culture, namely sexual identity, the ownership and commercial exploitation of the body, and the political power of medical institutions (Turner 1984, 1992, 1995a). The issues that now dominate medical sociology are central to society as a whole because medicine as an institution is crucial to modern systems of science, political power, and economic wealth. In this study of medical institutions, "the health care state" (Moran 1999) is useful as a perspective on the global medicoeconomic institutions of production and consumption of health. In this exposition, I shall explore the relationship between medicine and sexual identity and conclude with a discussion of the global exchange of organs, organ transplantation, and organ donation. The linking theme between the medical economy of organs and sexual identity is the importance of the sociology of the body in an understanding of medical science in its global environment.

In contemporary societies, sexual identity has become increasingly ambiguous. With the modernization of societies, there have been important legal changes resulting in greater, if reluctant, tolerance of homosexuality, gender-bending, cross-dressing, transsexualism, and sexual reassignment through surgery (Lewins 1995). The complexity of our sexual identities has also been underlined by the AIDS crisis, which has produced new forms of consciousness—indeed, a modern self (Rinken 2000). Medicine has historically exercised enormous power over legal decisions about how individuals are allocated gender positions. Medical institutions and medical beliefs have played a particularly important role in the social definition of the differences between homosexual and heterosexual identity, especially in the determination of ambiguous categories (Foucault 1980a). Although there have been important changes in public opinion about sexual identity, medical power remains closely associated with male control over the sexuality of women. Patriarchal power persists because historically the reproductive capacity of women has been a necessary basis for the inheritance and reproduction of property. The stable redistribution of family property through inheritance meant that successful biological reproduction was a necessary requirement of successful economic reproduction. Medical practice was closely harnessed to the maintenance of the traditional family, routine divisions between male and female, and conventional forms of the division of labor. Medical advice about "women's complaints," masturbation in young men, successful reproductive coitus, effective modes of female delivery, and the management of children were an important repertoire of the "family doctor." Medicine has therefore played an important part in shaping the sexual identities of men and women through the regulation of the body. We can gain an insight into the traditional role of medicine by looking at the treatment of those health conditions that appear to be peculiar to women.

In order to understand medical history, we need to understand the production of sexualities. The discourse of disease and illness was organized around the need to regulate bodies within a social and psychic framework in which the body was thought to be out of control. In the process of understanding sexuality historically and sociologically, we need to question naive interpretations of sexuality, which present modern society in terms of growing intimacy, expanding sexual pleasure, and the increasing importance of companionate marriage. From the perspective of Foucault, "sexuality" cannot be taken to be a naturally occurring or stable phenomenon. Within this Foucauldian framework, we need to understand the construction of sexualities as a plural, complex, and heterogeneous phenomenon.

While historically homosexuality has been a general feature of human societies, the eighteenth century produced "the homosexual" as a separate and distinct type of person and hence created a specific sexual identity, one that had to be isolated and then condemned by the official heterosexual sociopolitical regime. Medical science was crucial to this historical development. Thus the social history of heterosexuality is characterized by the emergence of the dominant male and mandatory marriage. More people were encouraged to define themselves in terms of a polar sexuality that was dependent on finding the opposite sex physically attractive. Heterosexual procreative and penetrative sex became the only permissible type of genital contact (Hitchcock 1997). This type of penetrative relationship is defined as phallocentric. Alongside this medical emphasis on penetration was the norm of female sexual passivity and the idea that male sexuality was rampant and difficult to control. Lesbian behavior was almost ignored because it did not and could not involve "real" penile penetration. By contrast, rape and sodomy were condemned. In fact, the antisocial character of penetrative sexual deviance was associated in popular culture with luxury and elite corruption, and given the dominance of the Protestant establishment, it was also associated with the spread of Catholicism. Court sodomy, homosexuality, rape, and incest were seen as the inevitable consequences of the corruption of society by the papacy. English society witnessed a significant increase in repressive legislation designed to curb sexual license, such as the Bawdy House Act of 1752. Church societies and voluntary associations, such as the Proclamation Society and the Society for the Suppression of Vice, were based on an ideology of women as victims of the unregulated sexual desire of men. The aim of legislation and church regulation was to keep women within the safe confines of the household. Medicine increasingly provided the scientific justification for these normative religious views of the nature of sexuality.

Women, Weight, and Wealth

Critical feminist theory in medical sociology and the history of medicine has argued that medical theories about sexuality reflected the prevailing view of women as frail and thus in need of male protection and, in cases of obvious deviance, regulation. The history of gynecology, as represented in medical textbooks, embraces the dominant social values, in which women's sexuality was regarded as either a mystery or a problem (Scully and Bart 1978). Historically, sexual dysfunction in gynecology textbooks has been a female, not male, problem. The medical ideology of female frailty simultaneously solved two issues: the disqualification of women as medical practitioners and their qualification as lay patients (Ehrenreich and English 1973). In practice, these various explanations and perspectives converged on one issue: disorders were associated with low social status and the absence of power, while medical doctrines, because they reflected dominant values, expressed and reinforced existing hierarchies of social control. The professional development of medicine has been closely associated with patriarchal culture, where the sexuality of women has been fundamental to the definition of female problems, both moral and medical (Clarke 1983).

Female complaints can be regarded as psychosomatic expressions of, and social responses to, the emotional problems built into the division of the social world into a public arena of authority and a private world of emotion and sensibility (Brumberg 1988). These ailments are illustrations of what Arthur Kleinman (1988, 57) has called "somatization," or "the communication of personal and interpersonal problems in a physical idiom of distress and a pattern of behavior that emphasizes the seeking of medical help." It is difficult to make a clear distinction between physical and mental health with a variety of health conditions that express powerlessness. For example, while agoraphobia (fear of public spaces) as a diagnostic label purports to describe a psychological disorder, it was expressive of Victorian morality, in which the good woman was a woman secluded within a household. Agoraphobia expressed an anxiety about sexual aggression or seduction in public spaces outside the household. These diagnostic notions can be regarded as retrospective and defensive, however, since the agoraphobic label emerged in Europe in a period when middle-class women were already beginning to leave the safety of the home as workers and professional employees. The label was paradoxically an attempt to secure women within traditional roles while recognizing their entry into the masculine spaces of work and employment.

In the modern period, anorexia nervosa has become preeminently attached to women. Like hysteria and agoraphobia, anorexia was seen to be predominantly a disorder of young women (Palmer 1980; Kalucy, Crisp, and Harding 1977). The onset of anorexia occurs at about age fifteen, and the majority of cases are clinically identified prior to age twenty-five. The condition is concentrated in the period of puberty and sexual development. There is historical evidence that the diagnostic label became increasingly popular among medical professionals in the 1970s, suggesting an increased prevalence of the illness (Crisp, Palmer, and Kalucy 1976). In 1945, when Ludwig Binswanger chronicled the case of Ellen West, he referred to anorexia as a new symptom, and in 1973 Hilde Bruch described anorexia as rare. By the 1980s, it was estimated that one in every two hundred women between the ages of thirteen and twenty-two suffered from the condition. Somewhere between 12 percent and 33 percent of American college women control their weight by vomiting, diuretics, and laxatives (Bordo 1993, 140).

The condition itself is physiologically, psychologically, and socially complex, and the symptoms of the disorder are diverse and varied. They include amenorrhea, lanugo, bradycardia, bulimia, and vomiting. Because weight loss and disturbed menstruation are part of the syndrome of anorexic women, clinical psychologists have favored a broader category for this type of disease, "dietary chaos syndrome" (Palmer 1979). Other medical research indicates that we should emphasize the psychological criteria of diagnosis, however, drawing attention to the fear of fatness and the pursuit of thinness as important features of the disorder (Bruch 1978). A distorted body image is an important element in the psychology of the condition. From a social psychological perspective, anorexia represents a control paradox, which can also be understood in religious terms as a type of asceticism in which there is a personal struggle to achieve spirituality through the management of the body. Researchers have drawn a parallel between medieval asceticism and the modern condition of anorexia in which the anorexic seeks a release from the profane world. Catherine J. Garrett (1996) argues that while medicine has invested a great deal in the diagnosis of anorexia, it has been less successful in, or concerned by, the discovery of processes of psychological recovery. Anorexic patients are often critical of the official diagnostic labels of psychiatry because they do not sympathetically address the patient's sense of self-loathing and existential suffering. Recovery requires effective rituals that will allow the patient to see anorexia as a spiritual quest and provide means to reenter society.

The critical literature on the anorexic condition has been significantly influenced by feminist theory, which treats the disorder as a consequence of women's subordinate position in society due to the sexual division of labor and patriarchal power (Caskey 1986). Women are caught in a contradictory set of expectations concerning their beauty, their social value, and their moral character (Chernin 1981). The disorder also has important symbols relating to the contradictory character of sexuality in young women. Autobiographical accounts give some indication that excessive slimming in puberty is connected with a rejection of adult sexuality through the suppression of menstruation. Overmuch obedience to parental control in order to achieve moral security is part of the drive to control their emotions in a period of their lives when these young women begin to form their first mature encounters and alliances with men (Bruch 1988). Furthermore, since consumer culture places a great emphasis on being slim, there are strong social pressures to control the body (Orbach 1978). The competition among siblings for parental attention is also a feature of the contradictory world of anorexia (J. Mitchell 2000). While conforming to the social norm of the slim body, the anorexic also suppresses her sexuality by the suppression of menstruation, which results from excessive dietary control. It is sociologically interesting to note that ballerinas, who in many respects encapsulate the modern notions of fitness, glamour, and sexual attractiveness, are particularly susceptible to anorexic pressures. Gelsey Kirkland, a famous American ballerina, was the epitome of balletic beauty, but in *Dancing on My Grave* (1986) she describes how her celebrity status eventually brought her drug dependency, anorexia, and personal crisis.

The contradictory nature of anorexia is precisely encapsulated in the title of Bruch's book *The Golden Cage* (1978), by which metaphor Bruch described the middle-class, overprotected, inward-looking, expressively charged family caught by the pressures of consumerism and social achievement. In this type of controlling family, anorexia is an expression of adolescent dissatisfaction with parental management. The young woman asserts her individuality in the face of powerful conventions and adult norms represented by her mother and her typically absent father. There is a contradictory relationship in the anorexic condition because the emphasis on competition and individual achievement in the middle-class family requires a high degree of personal independence with respect to the outer world. At the same time, the "good girl" owes obedience, subordination, self-control, and compliance to her mother. Regulation of diet and control of body size represent immediate and personal areas within which the young woman can express self-government and personal authority. Faced with the possibility of a disastrous failure at school or in her early career, the young woman may choose the sick role of anorexia as a solution to her sexual, social, and moral dilemmas.

Although anorexia nervosa can be understood in psychoanalytic terms as the struggle of young women against parental authority, in a more general sense anorexia, like nineteenth-century hysteria, expresses the social limitations of women within a society characterized by inequality between the sexes. Susan Bordo (1993, 141) recommends that we "take the psychopathologies that develop within a culture, far from being anomalies or aberrations, to be characteristic expressions of that culture; to be, indeed, the crystallization of much that is wrong with it."

Agoraphobia is an illness that resembles anorexia in its psychological and social dimensions. It, too, has been particularly prevalent among women. Approximately 89 percent of agoraphobics are female (Davidson 2000), probably because fear of open spaces reflects women's anxieties about the representation of their bodies in social space. In a culture that breeds such anxieties, medical discourse instructs women morally to take up social roles deemed suitable to their contradictory social status. The weight of a woman is particularly significant in this

cultural contradiction. The obese woman is out of control because the unrestrained and unregulated body is indicative of
moral weakness. To control women's bodies is to control their
personalities, and this authority over the body echoes a general
political process, which attempts to regulate competitive male-
female relations under a system of perpetual patriarchal power.

As the social status and citizenship rights of women begin
to approximate those of men (especially in employment, education, and welfare), the social behavior of men and women will
converge. Hence, their health characteristics will show similar
patterns of development. There is some evidence of gender convergence in both mental and physical disorders. In terms of
mental health, evidence from the United States suggests that
the traditional disparity between men and women has been reduced in the postwar period (Mumford 1983). In areas of deviance and criminality, which traditionally have been associated
with men, women have been increasingly involved. Throughout the industrial Western world, higher rates of alcoholism
among women have been reported in recent years. In some
areas of Britain, female admissions to programs for alcoholism
are almost as high as male admissions. Alcohol problems appear to increase as women seek greater social equality through
employment and competition. Generally speaking, the greater
the length of education, the lower the level of tobacco and alcohol consumption, but in Britain, women in the top civil
service hierarchy smoke and drink more than their male colleagues (Marmot and Davey Smith 1997). From a sociological
perspective, alcoholism is a condition that shows how women
are deviating from the conventional female role and adopting
masculine social characteristics in their attitudes and behavior.

In terms of smoking, as men were reducing their dependency on cigarettes in the middle of the twentieth century, women were increasing theirs. An alternative perspective is that precisely because women are subordinated, they tend to emulate the behavior of the dominant group.

The gender difference in smoking is now less pronounced, but women are experiencing a sharp increase in lung cancer. Because there is a time lag between smoking in adolescence and the onset of lung cancer, it was not until the 1980s and 1990s that epidemiologists noted a large increase in the incidence of lung cancer in women (Waldron 1991, 2000; Waldron and Lye 1989).

Recent research has suggested that the gender differential in health outcomes has been changing as more women enter the labor force and as more men experience instability in the labor market because of casual employment, unemployment, and early retirement (Annandale and Hunt 2000; Gove and Geerken 1977; McDonough and Walters 2001). What emerges from this research is the Durkheimian theme of the negative health consequences of social isolation. The poor health of women in traditional domestic roles is a function of their social isolation and lack of self-esteem, but as men in a modern economy also begin to experience the negative effects of social isolation and exclusion, differences between men and women begin to disappear (Graham 1984). Unemployed and unemployable men no longer enjoy the psychological benefits of the dignity of labor, and their self-respect declines as their status as gainfully employed citizens evaporates (Sennett 2003, 57).

Historically, body weight has been an important aspect of self-respect, and it is important, therefore, to examine the relationships between body weight by gender and weight norms over time. Comparative data on body size and weight show that growing affluence has increased body weight, as measured by the body mass index. Given the emphasis on slim bodies as a norm of sexual attractiveness, these social changes have produced an interesting paradox: as actual weight has gone up, cultural norms of desired weight have gone down. Between 1970 and 1990, obesity in Britain rose to about 17 percent, and in America almost 20 percent of men and 25 percent of women were obese. There are important variations by social class and gender, too: in lower social classes, one finds the highest consumption of "junk food." The traditional working classes survived on bulk food, such as potatoes and cabbage, but in a modern consumer society the working-class diet leans toward the consumption of snacks, alcohol, and sweets. In terms of gender, while 23 percent of men in the United States are dieting, 40 percent of women are attempting to lose weight.

The causes of increasing obesity are many: lack of exercise, dependence on fast food, and dining out. In a comparative study of U.S. and U.K. body-weight trends, Avner Offer (2001) has observed that the trends present a puzzle for sociological theory. Norbert Elias (1978) argues that with a growth in civilization there is a growth in self-control. With growing affluence in Europe and North America, however, self-control as measured by rising obesity is declining. Offer's explanation points to sexual competition and a sex-ratio imbalance. There is evidence from the sociology of courtship that slim women have more dates than fat women. Similarly, tall women tend to marry men of a higher socioeconomic standing. To compete in the marriage market, it is important for women to control their bodies through dieting. In marriage or other stable relationships, women with children put on weight, perhaps because they are no longer in a competitive relationship. In the postwar period, especially between the 1960s and 1980s, women looking for older males were in a decisively imbalanced competitive market. There is evidence, however, that those who practice periodic or excessive weight control face the long-term consequence of becoming overweight. Aggressive dieting tends to be associated with binging. The same pattern is repeated in anorexia, because anorexic women are also likely to suffer from bulimia. This sexual competition has driven down cultural norms of the slim body, while eating habits associated with fast-food restaurants have increased actual body weight.

Therefore, there is a complex relationship between sexual competition, body size, and health because there is a close relationship between obesity and illness, especially heart disease and diabetes. For example, working-class women have poor health and little competitive advantage in the sexual or marital market. Indulgences in junk food, alcohol, and smoking can be seen as emotional compensation for social disadvantage. This competitive market also has consequences for men. Romantic love in modern societies is contradictory because it celebrates both erotic, intense, fleeting romances and enduring, permanent, faithful love. These contradictions result from the transformation of love in the twentieth century through the growth of mass consumption and the association of romance and consumerism established by the mass media. While in America emotional commitment has been regarded since the eighteenth century as a necessary component of a successful marriage, it was not until the development of mass consumerism and advertising in the 1930s that a new emphasis on self-expression, romantic attachments, and adventure emerged in the marketplace. The "love utopia" (Illouz 1997) was based on a democratization of love and the possibility of mass consumption. "Love for everyone" was combined with "consumption for all." Social reality constantly brought this utopia into question, however. In the early decades of the twentieth century, marriage as an institution was in a profound crisis. The underlying factors were changes in matrimonial legislation, the entry of women into the labor force, unrealistic expectations about the romantic character of marriage and conflicts over domestic expenditure. Marriage-guidance experts began to devise practical solutions to inject fun into marriages because it was assumed that the companionate marriage was no longer adequate unless it could find space for erotic love and enjoyment.

BIOLOGY, SOCIETY, AND BIOPOLITICS

Medicine and medical authority continue to play a critical role in political debates about appropriate social roles for men and women, for example, in the contemporary controversies over homosexual men in the army and women in combat. Sexual identity in modern society has become more ambiguous and more open to a certain degree of negotiation. What is the possible extent of this negotiation of self in society? Medical innovations in technology have created new opportunities for reproduction. For example, couples may now reproduce after the death of one or both partners by storing their eggs and sperm. Artificial reproduction has expanded the possibility of fertility to infertile couples and elderly women, and medical technology provides the means for parents to select the sex of their children. These changes in the means by which, and the conditions under which, we reproduce inevitably bring about the transformation of familial and kinship relations. Because the social identity of people (who they are) is connected necessarily with where they come from (in kinship terms), these transformations in the possibilities of reproduction may eventually transform the processes by which we acquire identity. Ethics and medicine become entwined in complex and problematic patterns.

The cloned sheep Dolly brought media attention to the existence of innovative processes in biological sciences that have major implications for the ways in which societies operate. Cloning is simply one aspect of a revolution that has taken place in the applications of biological science to food production, reproduction, and medical procedures. Cloning is part of a larger set of issues about the relationship between society, medical science, and reproduction. While the first documented case of clinical artificial insemination of a human subject was in 1884, the first live-born child conceived through embryo transfer was in 1977. By 1989, it was estimated that 9,125 births were the result of artificial reproduction, rising to 50,000 by the mid-1990s. New reproductive techniques raise major legal issues about who has a right to reproduce, and thus these methods are fundamental to the growth of reproductive citizenship. Many societies leave reproductive decisions to gynecologists and their childless patients, as in the United States, while other societies have created extensive legislation to monitor and regulate reproduction. In Britain, reproductive techniques have permitted women in their late fifties to reproduce (Warnock

2002). The emergence of the geriatric mother has given greater urgency to the ethical question, is the right to reproduce universal?

In many respects, cloning can be seen as an extension of issues related to reproduction. While many governments are uncertain and concerned about the dramatic implications of human cloning, the idea of "therapeutic cloning" is attractive but may be, as it were, the back door to human cloning. Therapeutic cloning employs animal or human tissue to clone whole organs, such as hearts, lungs, and kidneys, that can be used in therapeutic organ transplants. Human embryo stem-cell research holds out the possibility of discovering cures for diabetes, Parkinson's disease, and Alzheimer's disease. But such research has been condemned by many, including the U.S. Conference of Catholic Bishops, who lobbied the U.S. Congress to block funding because it is seen as the first step toward human cloning. Stem-cell research, which deals with the fundamental cells that produce our basic organs, looks beneficial, but many Christians fear that it is impossible to prevent therapeutic cloning from becoming the slippery slope toward human cloning.

Biomedical research and genetic research more generally comprise an expanding section of the global economy. In order to make this research profitable, corporations have entered into a growing legal conflict over the patenting of segments of the human genetic code. In October 1999, the U.S. company Celera Genomics announced that it had decoded one-third of the human genome blueprint and would seek patents to protect its intellectual property. The competition among such global corporations for profits from genetic research can contradict one of the basic principles of science: the free flow of information within the scientific community. It also conflicts with the formation and development of national science policies. These developments will shape the evolution of science and produce new areas of research interest, including the development of global competition for patents on genetic material, conflicts between profitability and freedom of information, the creation of legal frameworks within which national policies on biomedical research can evolve, and the development of legal and social frameworks for new reproductive technologies.

New reproductive technologies are an important topic for sociologists because they can change the nature and functions of kinship relationships. The essential feature of these technologies is that they separate sexual intercourse from biological reproduction and hence bring into question the traditional roles of husbands and wives, fathers and mothers, as necessary social roles in reproduction. These technologies make possible a range of new social relationships in reproductive arrangements. For example, donations of egg and sperm may be from people who have died, and hence a viable child may be born to biological parents who are not viable because they are already deceased. The new technologies open up possible social relations that go well beyond surrogacy and adoption. When science separates sex and reproduction, it is difficult to determine who is the mother. Is the mother the donor of the egg, the surrogate mother who carries and delivers, or the parent who brings up and cares for the child? In some countries, such as Italy, where women over age sixty have reproduced using the new technologies, it is unclear who will take responsibility for the maintenance of the child. It is not inconceivable that medical scientists could construct an artificial womb that would allow a homosexual male couple to reproduce without the assistance of a surrogate mother. In the long run, one can imagine a society in which men with womb implants could reproduce successfully without female assistance. New technologies are creating possibilities for new family relationships, but these changes are not effectively regulated by law or professional consensus.

The tensions in British legislation and policy on reproduction are an important illustration of these issues. Because childless couples in Britain may have to wait two years to secure an egg, they are making use of the Internet to find egg donors. The sale of eggs in the United States has also become big business. Donor agencies advertise for eggs in Ivy League student newspapers, and up to fifty thousand dollars has been offered for preferred characteristics in ethnic background, height, and intellectual aptitude. In the United Kingdom, the Human Fertilisation and Embryology Authority attempts to regulate access to eggs. In the United States market forces primarily determine donation. Where there is little state or professional regulation, reproductive relationships resemble a free market in which eggs and sperm are exchanged like other commodities. The result is to increase what we might call a system of reproductive inequality.

State regulation of health raises complex issues relating to human freedom in a liberal society. In Britain, for example, in August 1999, the local authorities in the Camden district in North London attempted to compel a couple to have their baby tested because the mother was HIV positive. The parents opposed the council on the grounds that the child would be stigmatized by a compulsory test and that the state has no right to regulate family life. The council's legal argument was that the state has the capacity to override parental wishes where it is acting in the best interests of the child.

The social consequences of cloning, genetics, and new reproductive technologies will be revolutionary, and the conflicts that will emerge from the new biology, in policy formation, politics, and law, will be profound. There is an important area of comparative and legal research on government responses to genetic research and patent policy. Who will own the human body? Already this question has become significant in the area of organ transplants and reproduction, and debates will become extensive as new medical procedures become possible. The fundamental problem is the changing relationship between the self, the body, and society. Medical technology and microbiology hold the promise (through the Human Genome Project, cloning, transplants, "wonder drugs," and microsurgery) of freedom from aging, disability, and death. Cosmetic surgery promises us beautiful bodies, if not eternal youth. These medical possibilities have given rise to utopian visions of a world wholly free from disease—a new mirage of health. It is clear that the human body will come to stand in an entirely new relationship to self and society as a result of these technological developments. These medical changes will have major consequences for family life, reproduction, work, and aging. They also raise important issues for the ownership and use of the human body. Should people be free to sell parts of their bodies for commercial gain? Furthermore, these changes create opportunities for the development of a global medical system of governance in which medicine may exercise an expanded power over life and death. Few national governments have attempted to regulate this global medical system through legislation.

SOVEREIGN POWER AND THE BODY

We have the possibility of creating, or at least cloning, life through medical science. We also have the power to destroy it. Although the majority of governments are hostile to the formal and explicit development of a policy of eugenics, all governments have formal but largely implicit eugenics policies in terms of legislation on marriage, abortion, adoption, and reproduction. Governments continue to worry about the adoption of formal eugenics because of the legacy of eugenics policies in Nazi Germany (Weindling 1989). It is also clear, however, that doctors operate with de facto eugenics practices. The philosopher Peter Singer has controversially pointed to the inconsistency in social policies that support abortion but reject euthanasia, and he has criticized the wisdom of medical ethics that embrace "sanctity of life" as an overriding principle. In the controversial issue of severely handicapped children, Singer (1979) argues that it has been found that doctors and nurses, when confronted with such children, employ a practice of "selective nontreatment" that constitutes implicit infanticide. Selective nontreatment is a principle of moral queuing. Such medical practices are based on a principle of quality of life rather than sanctity of life. When a child's impairment will severely preclude his or her enjoyment of any reasonable quality of life, doctors may adopt selective nontreatment to permit the child to die with minimal pain and loss of dignity. These arguments about quality directly challenged the position adopted

by President Ronald Reagan to enforce sanctity-of-life policies in U.S. hospitals. The evidence produced by Singer in his
controversial *Rethinking Life and Death* (1994) suggests that
sanctity-of-life policies have failed.

The moral dilemmas that have been explored in Singer's
"practical ethics" can be seen within a broader context that
amounts to what we may call the industrialization of the body.
The commercial use of the human body invites us to adopt
the critical political-economy view of society as a medical-
industrial complex because the body can be broken down into
parts that become commodities. Many of the related social
changes have their roots in commercial applications of genetic
research, but perhaps a more dramatic and emotive illustration
of commercialization is the world market in kidney sales from
poor to rich countries. This sale is controversial in that its sup-
porters argue that it provides immediate cash benefits to the
donating family while the sick receive a much-needed organ.
Critics of the system argue that organs typically come from
women in poor communities and go to men in rich societies.
The women do not receive adequate medical support after donation and often suffer from infections and exhaustion, and the
costs of drugs to suppress the immune systems of recipients
represents a significant economic burden on recipient families
(Scheper-Hughes 2001a).

Organ donation is in formal terms voluntary, but in practice
kidney donation is a response to extreme poverty. Poor Indian
women often sell a kidney in order to feed their children. Donations have not always been voluntary. Before the end of
apartheid, human tissues and organs were harvested from
people in intensive-care units without the knowledge of their

33333333

families (Scheper-Hughes 2001b). These practices raise difficult moral and practical questions about whether a free market in body parts truly exists. The sale of body parts and their legal framework again provoke a fundamental question: who owns the body?

Global markets in organs have been of considerable interest to both anthropologists and sociologists, who have generally been critical of organ sales and bioharvesting in remote aboriginal communities. It is for this reason that therapeutic cloning would be a significant medical advance and probably end the market in human organs. These medical developments point conclusively to the continuity of third world poverty and dependency, however, and to the fact that medical improvements in the developed world are unlikely to help third world societies until basic social and economic improvements take place: the growth of per capita income and improvement in basic services, such as sewer systems, clean water, adequate diet, education, and shelter.

In this discussion of the body as property, the concept of governmentality is useful as a general analytical framework. The term governmentality emerged in Foucault's later writing on the state and administration, namely, in his thesis that the modern state's primary concern is no longer with the punishment of the criminal body but with its productive capacities (1991). The idea behind Bentham's reform of punishment was to make the body useful rather than to punish it. The analysis of governmentality rests more generally on Foucault's historical commentaries on the body in Western society. In his *History of Sexuality* (1979, 139–40), the relationship between power, body, and government is explicit in his argument that the regulation of the human body was first ensured by a variety of new disciplines ("an anatomo-politics of the human body") and by an array of regulatory controls ("a bio-politics of the population"). The concept of "population" as part of demographic science was originally an important indicator of the state's administrative interest in making populations fully productive in economic and social terms. Notions about the productive capacities of society became important only in the course of the development of modern political institutions. In Foucault's political philosophy, disciplinary power such as Bentham's panopticism functions to produce servile, disciplined, and effective bodies through a micropolitics of disciplinary regimes, practices, and regulations. Docile but productive bodies are functional for the modern state as part of a general apparatus of control or governmentality (Foucault 1980a). The modern individual who is disciplined and exercises self-control arose from these political and administrative changes to the organization of the state. The exercise of power in the modern state is typically local, diffuse, practical, and normative.

Governmentality had three aspects (Foucault 1991, 102–3). First are the institutions, procedures, calculations, and tactics that permit the exercise of this specific form of power. Human population is its target, political economy is its principal form of knowledge, and apparatuses of security are its essential technical means. Second, there is the formation of a series of specific government apparatuses and the development of a complex of *savoirs*. Finally, there were a number of historical processes by which the medieval state of justice, converted into the administrative state during the fifteenth and sixteenth centuries, gradually emerged as governmentality.

Governmentality has become the common foundation of modern forms of political rationality. For example, the administrative systems of the state have been extended in order to maximize the state's productive control over the processes of the population. More specifically, the conceptualization of population marked the origin of the administrative sciences. With the demographic upswing in Europe, it was necessary to produce a system of measurement, surveillance, and control. Modern medicine lies at the core of this political system of governance.

Governmentality is the generic term for these power relations. Historically, the power of the state has been less concerned with sovereignty over possessions (land and wealth) and more concerned with maximizing the productive power of administration over population and reproduction. One implication of Foucault's theory of power is that over time, power relations tend to become more refined, detailed, and specific. Whereas simple forms of patriarchal power took the whole body as its site of operation, the modernization of the state and medical science has involved an increasing differentiation of the body. Medical power itself has become specialized through the differentiation of the body into its respective parts. The body of modern medicine has thus been differentiated into the specialized sites of the medical gaze and medical science. Hospitals have consequently focused not only on particular bodies—such as the children's hospital—but on specific parts of the body—the eye hospital or the ear, nose, and throat clinic.

These specialized and differentiated forms of medicine are not punitive divisions. They seek to make the body more productive, as Foucault would argue, by forcing the body to reveal its secrets. Foucault interpreted the exercise of administrative power in productive terms, enhancing population potential through, for example, state support for the family. The state's involvement in and regulation of reproductive technology is an important example of governmentality, in which the desire of couples to reproduce is enhanced by the state's support of new technologies. The demand for fertility is supported by a pro-family ideology that regards the normal household as a reproductive social space. In modern society, childlessness is regarded as a calamity, or at least a problem for which modern medicine has a cure. The childless woman is somebody who has failed to enter adult society successfully.

This extension of administrative rationality was first concerned with the demographic processes of birth, morbidity, and death and later with the psychological health of the population. Medical practice in the eighteenth century recognized an important connection between the government of the body through dietary management and the government of society through effective political management (Turner 1992, 1996, 1997c). Political theory saw the necessary connections between the ownership and control of bodies and the sovereignty of the state.

The question of the ownership of the body cannot be disconnected, therefore, from the problem of sovereignty of the state. In traditional political systems, women, children, and servants generally were conceptualized as part of the household, over which the male head of the household had absolute legal rights. Economy was simply the management of a household, within which a woman was regarded as an economic asset. When applied to kingship, this legal doctrine supported absolutism but was challenged by individualistic notions of private property and the limited right of kings to rule under a social contract. The bourgeois theory of property as the investment of labor depended on a distinction between ownership and control of property and rights to its use.

There are important differences in issues relating to the exploitation of the sexual labor of another (prostitution), ownership of other persons' bodies for the sake of economic production (slavery), and sale of parts of a body for commercial gain (the organ market). At the core of the contemporary legal debate about bodies are notions of self-ownership and consent, but scientific developments have opened up economic opportunities for the commercial exploitation of the human body. In particular, modern genetic sciences have stimulated another set of possibilities, namely, the development of patents on genetic innovations. We are at the beginning of a new phase in the evolution of scientific medicine—the global harvesting, commodification, and sale of genetic codes and genetic material.

The problem of the body needs to be made more explicit in any reading of social and political theory. The body is central to any theory of power and to any modern vision of citizenship and human rights. Under conditions of chattel slavery, bodies were typically the property of the state in a system of absolute power. Modern individualism, norms of social equality, and democratization have made the unconditional ownership of another's body unlikely, and thus modern consumption of sexual services involves a rental charge more than ownership. The patrimonial state, in the form of a sovereign, naturally assumed rights over the whole bodies of persons, but the modern state encounters a range of different issues. With advances in medical science (particularly anatomy and anaesthetics), it became possible for a global market to emerge in the sale and exchange of parts of bodies. With the further differentiation of the body into what can be called suborganic particles, there are new possibilities for the commercialization of the body through the sale of patents on the genetic code.

REPRODUCTIVE CITIZENSHIP

The growth of modern citizenship is closely associated with governmentality in terms of disciplining the subject. Because gender is crucially important to the production of modern subjectivity, we need to consider the relationship between body, sexuality, reproduction, and the state. Recent writing in citizenship studies has underlined the neglect of gender in the analysis of the national development of citizen entitlements and obligations in the nation-state. We need to extend the discussion of citizenship, nationalism, and gender by examining the relationship between parenthood and entitlement. Reproducing the next generation of citizens through marriage and household formation is a central means of acquiring comprehensive entitlements of citizenship and fulfilling its corresponding obligations.

Contemporary government policies on new reproductive technologies implicitly demonstrate the general importance of eugenics for the modern state. Because the majority of Western societies enjoy only modest rates of successful reproduction in demographic terms, the state promotes the desirability of fertility as a foundation of social participation. Recent debates about the decline of the birth rate in post-Communist societies are instructive in terms of the state's relationship to population stagnation in a society in crisis. For example, the Russian birth rate has fallen from 1.89 children per woman in 1990 to 1.17 in 2000, and it is predicted that the population of the Russian Federation will decline from 147 million to 123 million by 2015. Alcoholism and drug abuse have had a dramatic impact on the health of young men, while poverty and the collapse of public health institutions are associated with the rise of tuberculosis and AIDS. Abortions in Russia are four times higher than in the United States, or one for every thirty-five people in the country. In 2003, legal changes restricted the grounds for abortion, which is now permissible if the woman's health is at risk or in cases of rape. While President Vladimir Putin has promised to reverse these population trends—for example, by the repatriation of ethnic Russians—the ultranationalist Vladimir Zhirinovsky has proposed that the family code be amended to legitimize polygamy. Although the Russian dilemma (an increasing death rate and a declining birth rate) is unusual in a technologically sophisticated society, it underlines the relationship between the state, governmentality, and demography.

Governments of the developed world are consequently concerned with the "failure" of heterosexual households to achieve reproduction. The privileged position given to heterosexuality is a function of how public policies seek to normalize reproduction as the desired outcome of marriage. While more women are acquiring a university education in Britain and America, women who have been educated to the degree level are 50 percent more likely to remain childless than their uneducated peers. These developments have important implications for family life and citizenship in the educated middle classes. The liberal regime of modern citizenship regards parenthood in "normal" families, rather than heterosexuality, as the defining characteristic of the "average" citizen and as the basis for social entitlement. Reproduction through heterosexual intercourse has simply been, until recently, the only means to achieve the social, cultural, and biological goals of parenthood. The introduction of technologies of artificial human reproduction in the late 1970s underlined how reproduction plays a foundational role in citizenship. These technologies provide the potential for reproduction without heterosexual intercourse. Despite their widespread acceptance as a treatment for infertility, new reproductive technologies remain controversial as medical procedures. Since the late 1970s, methods of artificial human reproduction have produced considerable public anxiety because they promise innovative means of human fertilization and provide unanticipated options for family formation. The technologies explicitly raise the issues of mothering, parenthood, conception, and implicitly the nature of the self in modern society. Government responses to these technical and social challenges reveal the moral assumptions of the state toward parents and families, namely the system of reproductive values prevalent in society.

Gay and lesbian movements have claimed that sexual liberation, especially the right of individuals to decide on their own sexual orientation and sexual pleasures, is an important component of a civilized and egalitarian society (Bell and Binnie 2002). These arguments promote the idea of "sexual rights" as an important extension of the liberal model of social citizenship as a set of civil, political, and social rights (Evans 1993). The growth of such rights has been described as the early formation of "intimate citizenship" (Plummer 2000). In sociological terms, these changes in social attitudes form part of a larger "transformation of intimacy" (Giddens 1992). However, these accounts of sexual citizenship run into fundamental problems relating to individual rights.

There are three issues that theories of sexual or intimate citizenship must confront. First, critics of modern consumerism argue that rights to personal sexual activity are merely a new dimension of leisure activity that we might call hedonistic consumption; these rights to sexual pleasure have little to do with fundamental rights of personal freedom. Such rights to sexual fulfillment are better described as "consumer rights." Second, sexual rights appear to cover two rather separate issues: the demand of gay and lesbian individuals to enjoy the same rights as heterosexuals (sexual citizenship proper) and the expectation of increased sexual pleasure in a more open and liberal society (intimate citizenship). The rights of gay and lesbian individuals to equality under the law can be characterized as a citizenship claim. But intimate citizenship at best looks like an aspect of the negative liberty to enjoy a right provided that it does not inhibit the freedoms of other individuals (Berlin 1979, 122).

The state's interest in sexuality and sexual identity is secondary and subordinate to its primary demographic objective of securing and enforcing the historic connection between reproduction and citizenship. Reproductive citizenship as a concept is sociologically and legally more adequate than the idea of sexual citizenship. It recognizes the state's interest in population within the framework of governmentality. State building, nationalism, and reproductive citizenship are necessarily connected to reproduction when it is supported by traditional ideologies of patriarchy. The nation-state presupposes a continuing pattern of patriarchy and patriotism as the dual legacy of monarchy and state building. The modern system of nation, citizenship, and masculinity has been changed by the global challenge to national sovereignty, by the transformations of work and warfare in modern societies, and by the transformation of sexuality and parenthood associated with the development of reproductive technology. Despite these fundamental social and political changes, the foundation of national citizenship and the basis of individual entitlement remain legally and socially connected to heterosexual reproduction and, hence, to the nuclear family. A familial ideology of procreation has been a major legitimating support of the contemporary ensemble of entitlements that constitute the social rights of citizenship. One might say that the state's eugenic commandment is biblical: "Go forth and multiply."

NEW REPRODUCTIVE TECHNOLOGIES

The paradox of new reproductive technologies is that while they address what is regarded as a biological problem (infertility), they become enmeshed in complex social issues (abortion, medical power, unregulated markets, and confusion of values). For example, these technologies have helped to replace a unified concept of motherhood with diverse forms, such as genetic, gestational, and social motherhood. Public anxiety about the unintended consequences of the new genetics has raised contentious questions about the possibility and nature of the regulation of medicine and science in modern society. Conventional institutional mechanisms, such as professional autonomy, are no longer believed to be adequate, but regulation by market forces is unpredictable and almost certainly incompatible with many national policy goals. In short, the changing technologies of reproduction raise major problems for the women's movement, public policy, and traditional religious values relating to motherhood. These social changes have been especially acute for the Roman Catholic Church, which has remained officially opposed to any transformation of family life. Radical feminists who have opposed the technological intervention of medical science and technology in motherhood on the grounds that it is a form of patriarchy have often either implicitly or unintentionally defended motherhood as a "natural" event. The possibility that artificial wombs will become available to infertile couples is a challenge to "natural" motherhood. Those branches of feminism that have rejected technologically assisted reproduction are in danger of reproducing the conservative cultural assumptions that women are indeed natural creatures outside society while men and male science stand inside society. Because radical feminism has attacked unnatural scientific interventions, its position has some similarity with that of Catholic orthodoxy. It is often noted that there is a convergence of conservative religious women and radical feminists on the issues of pornography, abuse of women, and the negative consequences of medical science. These tensions in feminist theory are illustrated by the mid-1980s debates in the Feminist International Network on the New Reproductive Technologies (FINNRET) and the emergence of the Feminist International Network of Resistance to Reproductive and Genetic Engineering (FINNRAGE). Feminist concern with the negative impact of science on women's reproduction was expressed through metaphors such as "womb leasing," "egg farms," "living laboratories," and "breeding brothels," but these metaphors associated women with a guardianship of nature. The paradox of modern medical technology is that the more we are able to control the body, the greater the uncertainty we feel about what is natural about our bodies and what might be legitimate forms of medical intervention in them. The more we reduce the vulnerability of the body, the more we increase the precariousness of political institutions.

Clinical medical practice has typically evolved within an ethico-legal vacuum that in Europe did not come under public scrutiny until the mid-1990s. In this sense, policy formation has been retrospective and in the context of cultural subterfuge. The general framework for clinical therapeutic effort is a "narrative of hope," in which innovations are scientific breakthroughs, pioneering work, and medical successes. These medical developments have transformed infertility from reproductive incapacity (sterility) to a condition of potential reproductive capacity. Victorian "marital sterility" has been replaced or reconstructed as the infertility epidemic of the 1990s.

These apparently neutral scientific advances disguise deep-seated cultural assumptions about gender. For example, infertility has been defined as a female pathology despite the rhetoric of equivalence in the infertility health-promotion literature. Male infertility is treated as incidental or contributory; its cause is in the external environment, resulting from general pollution. Patient-information booklets avoid discussing biological pathology in male infertility. While new reproductive technologies may produce some medical successes, the low success rates are explained as an aspect of the inefficiency of natural reproductive waste. Reference to "one in six" couples suffering from infertility has become a taken-for-granted statistic in the popular debate and an important figure that legitimizes medical intervention. The metaphor of epidemic has had a powerful effect on debate.

The moratorium on in vitro fertilization (IVF) research in Britain between 1971 and 1978 was followed by a scientific rat race. There is now great uncertainty about the legitimate and therapeutic use of biomedical science, and the moral-political stalemate has allowed antiabortion lobbies to flourish alongside the questionable exploitation of human biology by commercial interests. The result is an unregulated movement in medical innovation that will produce wholly unknown and unanticipated outcomes in human reproduction. The growth of the bioethics discourse in the 1990s was a response to public anxiety about the social implications of new biological technologies, but such bioethics reports have tended to accept scientific and technical answers to value questions and to promote normative positions that are essentially retrospective (Fukuyama 2002).

The issue of contraception, IVF treatment, and reproductive technology has been particularly complex in Ireland, where it poses almost insoluble dilemmas for the Catholic hierarchy (McDonnell 2001). Physicians began assisted reproduction there in 1985, but a moratorium was quickly imposed and not lifted until 1987. Between 1985 and 1987, a consensus was established in the medical profession that accepted IVF for infertile married couples within a normal reproductive age group. One contradiction was the ethical ban on the use of donor sperm for IVF until 1998. This ethical stance prohibited the use of medical techniques in Ireland that were available elsewhere: gamete donation, surrogacy, IVF with donor sperm, and embryo freezing. The establishment of the National Infertility Support and Information Group (NISIG) in 1996 created an important patient-advocacy organization, but it also formalized the tension between conservative Catholic clinicians and a younger, more liberal generation. The tensions between public and private provision were important, and the expansion of the private sector made public regulation more difficult. The ethical prohibition on nonmarried couples in IVF programs became defunct.

A critical turning point occurred when an October 1996 television program discussed the clinical practice of disposing of spare embryos by placing them in a woman's cervix, thereby avoiding the problem of either storing or freezing the surplus embryos. Another cultural subterfuge was the rhetorical use of the expression *zygote freezing* to avoid the phrase *embryo freezing*. These contradictions and evasions resulted in legislation to create a state-regulated statutory register of clinicians. It also established a committee to advise the minister of health. The state's involvement raised acute questions about professional autonomy. The committee favored a voluntary licensing authority that would preserve professional autonomy, but the question of what should be left to clinical judgment remains contentious.

These scientific developments and ethical debates have raised an inescapable question about the nature of motherhood and the status of women. The possibility and the reality of the "postmenopausal birth phenomenon," in which European women as old as sixty-eight have been artificially impregnated, have raised an important issue about responsible parenting. It has become important for the legitimacy of the medical profession to normalize and naturalize the social implications of such radical deployment of the reproductive technology. While state regulation has been widely advocated, it is recognized that patient demand can always be satisfied in an open market by seeking assistance in other countries. One way around some of these difficulties has been to view the medical use of embryos to overcome infertility as analogous to the traditional practice of adoption.

CONCLUSION: LAW AND THE MODERN BODY

Legal regulation involves a system of values that conflicts with the market as a system of supply and demand. This conflict, between legal and economic regulation, is particularly problematic in the control of the scientific dismemberment of human bodies. The potential marketization of women's bodies by reproductive technologies was readily recognized by feminists (Corea 1985). The feminist diagnosis was prescient. Internet marketing of surrogate mothers and human gametes now spans the globe. The technology of the Internet promotes the globalization of the human-body market, which in turn was made possible by new reproductive technologies and presents the greatest challenge to any attempt to regulate the market through the imposition of moral standards upheld by law. The global market in human organs is, in Durkheim's terms, anomic. The next regulatory problem arising in this field is corporate control of genetic codes via patenting. Patents are important because they make the global sale of genetic information commercially viable, but they also ensure the economic inequalities between the developed and the developing worlds.

The revolution in microbiology and the application of genetic engineering to the body in contemporary society have raised new legal questions. Changes in the contemporary biological sciences and their commercial application invite us to make a distinction between three levels of embodiment for legal theory. In modern societies, law in principle will have to distinguish between rights: to whole bodies (in practice, to persons); to buy, sell, or store parts of bodies (as in organ transplants, donations, and sales and the commodification of human reproductive material—for example, eggs and sperm); and to explore and exploit what we might call information particles of bodies (such as DNA codes and genetic maps). This situation represents an important development, since modern science has made possible the commercial exploitation of bodily phenomena below the level of the whole organism.

The outright ownership of a whole person may appear to be an obsolete legal idea, but in reality the sale of women into sexual slavery in the societies of the former Soviet Union is a growing problem in Eastern Europe. Self-possession is still fundamental to liberal theory, but the tradition of possessive individualism from John Locke onward never envisioned the prospect of a rational person willingly selling a part of his or her body (a kidney, for instance) for profit. Globalization and commercialization have also had important consequences for the debate. For example, it is now possible for foreigners to buy the kidneys of executed convicts in China. *The Observer* in 2000 reported that rich customers from Melaka were paying ten thousand dollars in cash for kidneys from the People's Liberation Army Hospital in the provincial city of Chongqing, where it is alleged that condemned prisoners are allowed to die once their organs have been removed.

The commercial use of body parts and particles raises serious ethical questions that do not have neat solutions. The creation of human embryos in vitro and their storage in fertility clinics have made "latent" human bodies potentially available for experimentation and purchase. These technological developments of the early twenty-first century are forcing governments to impose legal regulations that attempt to protect human life (Warnock 1985; Mulkay 1997). Whether a conceptus is a body is contestable, but the delineation of its embodiment in principle is crucial to its treatment in practice. Organ transplant sales are not like the sale of other body parts, such as hair. The practice of selling human hair for a profit was not regarded as reprehensible in an era when wigs were fashionable. Within the framework of political economy, prostitution might be regarded as the alienation of labor or as the sale of the use of a body for commercial purposes, but since prostitutes are themselves typically controlled by male pimps, the issue of ownership and control is more complex. The real test of the notion of ownership may well lie in the question of how the law manages the regulation of the use of human reproductive material, such as sperm or gametes. Because transactions involving such material are typically regarded as having profound implications for the nature and meaning of life itself, many governments have not been content to allow the market to determine them. Given the potentially damaging unintended consequences of new reproductive technologies, cloning, organ sales, and genetic interventions, governments may attempt to impose governmentality or perhaps a new pattern of patriarchy. Past efforts to establish formal governmental regulation of the commercial arena of biomedical activity indicate that any attempt to impose effective, long-term regulation over the market is likely to fail. These commercial and medical developments are therefore likely to make our social environment more precarious and more risky.

Chapter Seven
HEALTH, RISK, AND GLOBALIZATION

INTRODUCTION: GLOBAL SOCIETY, HEALTH,
AND INFORMATION TECHNOLOGY

IN THE STUDY OF HEALTH AND ILLNESS IN modern society, the
new medical sociology comprehends medical institutions and
health and illness within the context of global processes. We
can no longer study the treatment of disease in an exclusively
national framework because the character of disease and its
treatment are global. Medical institutions and professions are
subject to global pressures, especially from insurance and funding arrangements. To take one obvious illustration, the ownership and current development of the pharmaceutical industry
are global. We are also on the verge of health-care systems that
will depend on global electronic communications and information systems. One remarkable example is telesurgery, which
involves the use of robot-assisted distance surgery. Telesurgi-
cal operations have to overcome a variety of problems, including long-distance transmission delays. Surgery has historically
evolved through its association with the military. The development of surgery—for example, by Ambroise Paré in his treatment of gunshot wounds in the sixteenth century—has been
driven by military conflict and the need to treat traumatic injuries sustained in combat. Telesurgery will make possible the

230

provision of rapid surgical support in global military campaigns. The consumer demand for health products is also increasingly organized through global economies. The healthy body is being promoted globally through fitness clubs and sports associations. Fitness Holdings, for example, is one of the world's largest health-club companies, with outlets in eleven countries, including Hong Kong, Sweden, and South Korea. In the United Kingdom, Fitness First, another fitness chain, has also expanded with the growth of global and domestic demand for healthy lifestyles.

However, health-care systems have often been slow to adopt innovations in information technology because the hardware and software are often insufficiently advanced to make a useful contribution to care. The value of telemedicine will vary considerably by medical specialism. For example, because clinical work in pulmonary medicine, neurology, and cardiology is still based on a physical examination and questioning of the patient, telecommunication is not seen to be important in that area (Lehoux et al. 2002). In the future, however, patients and doctors will be able to use broadband technologies to deliver health-care packages to homes and hospitals. The growth of e-health will create virtual hospitals, transform health education, and deliver health services to patients with limited mobility. E-health might also improve health delivery to remote communities. The technology and delivery systems for such innovations will necessarily be global, and they will be organized and owned by global health corporations.

In a period of global communication and transportation, disease does not recognize national borders. The 2003 outbreak of SARS, which spread rapidly from Beijing to Toronto, is a good example. The spread of infectious disease is also closely associated with the global conduct of war. The deadly Ebola virus is often carried through central Africa by guerrilla troops—for example, by the Lord's Resistance Army, a messianic rebel army that blends Christianity and Islam, and passed between southern Sudan and Uganda in 2003. The global spread of narcotics also has an important impact on national health statistics, through its negative effect on individual health behaviors. In America, the domestic politics of Colombia have a major outcome on health behavior in New York because the supply of drugs can be disrupted by domestic conflicts in South America. For the same economic and political reasons, the collection of the opium crop in Afghanistan and central Asia has a direct impact on health and lifestyle in London and Sydney. The rapid spread of crack cocaine as a lifestyle drug among young people, sex workers, and ethnic minority groups in inner cities in the last fifteen years has had detrimental consequences for health, especially in terms of enhanced HIV risk (A. Green, Day, and Ward 2000). Crack use has given rise to new forms of prostitution (sex for crack) among young women, who become socially stigmatized as "crack whores."

These global markets shape the health risks of Western urban cultures, but there is a still darker side to this discussion of medical globalization. Bioterrorism is now a major threat to modern states. Government concerns about the use of biological weapons have increased as a result of the sarin nerve-gas attack by a Japanese religious cult in 1995—which killed twelve and injured five thousand in Tokyo's subway system—and the anthrax attack in the United States in 2001. The U.S. Army has identified smallpox, anthrax, and botulism as organisms that can be easily disseminated in a civilian population. In order to understand the rapidly changing environment of health and illness, we need to look more closely at how social scientists analyze globalization and risk.

While the debate about personal identity in cultural postmodernity came to dominate much of the humanities and social sciences in the 1970s, two themes—risk society and globalization—have shaped contemporary academic and public discussion in the new millennium. To some extent, the multiplication of risks and the compression of social space have merged into a single issue, namely, the intensified precariousness of modern institutions. Globalization involves both a qualitative and a quantitative transformation of risk. As a result, the intensification of risk requires global regulation. Public interest in global processes has produced an important intellectual paradigm shift, in which the boundary between environment ("nature") and society ("culture") is contentious and problematic. Ulrich Beck's *Risk Society* (1992), first published in Germany in 1986, helped to transform a somewhat tired discussion of modernization and industrialization into a dynamic analysis of "late modernity," where "reflexive modernization" is the key process. In response, many sociologists have argued that the conventional theoretical paradigms of the social sciences have to be abandoned in order to grasp a new social reality based on global flows and networks rather than national societies. This new system of communication requires a "mobile sociology" (Urry 2000) that can discuss the end of "society" and the rise of a new social order based on networks, fluids, flows, complexity, and scapes. If modernization assumed that modern society would be well structured and orderly, then contemporary sociology understands late modernity through the lens of complexity and contingency. Global society in a deregulated global economy is supremely disorderly, as the attack on the World Trade Center on September 11, 2001, sadly demonstrated.

Of course, the concept of risk is hardly an original addition to the social sciences. Economics had its modern origin in the calculation of risk investment associated with long-distance trading relations during the rise of new colonies in the seventeenth century. Writing in the 1730s, Robert Cantillon, the author of *Essai sur la nature du commerce en général,* assumed a necessary relationship between risk and entrepreneurship and laid the foundations for the development of a more complete theory of capitalist risk-taking behavior, which developed into the economic sociology of Joseph Schumpeter (Higgs 1931). The notions of industrial hazards and the capitalist's capital risks were a central component of Karl Marx's political economy, which recognized industrial competition for profit as a principal mechanism of the destructive nature of capitalist accumulation. There were similar assumptions behind public health movements. As the 1840s investigations of Rudolf Virchow and Max von Pettenkofer show, hygienists and public health investigators clearly understood the generic health risks of early capitalism (Turner 2000a).

The study of risk has been a permanent feature of the scientific understanding of the capitalist economy. Beck's theory of risk, which grew out of his earlier work on industrial sociology, renewed this study through his innovative sociological view of the environmental debate in Germany; he showed that risks had become a generic feature of modernization. This sociological reflection on the environmental issue in terms of the contradiction between nature and society was quickly absorbed into mainstream sociological research (Eder 1996; Lash, Szerszynski, and Wynne 1996), but the more subtle and complex features of Beck's commentary on trust, expert opinion, and individualization have by comparison been less prominent in academic discussion.

The intellectual development of globalization theory is equally complex. It, too, has an established history and can be traced through the theory of the internationalization of politics and the growth of a world system in economics. Although aspects of the globalization process can be discovered in the internationalization of politics, we should not confuse the notions of international and global. Whereas international relations presuppose a system of nation-states, globalization theory attempts to understand global processes that are not directly grounded in nation-states. For example, it is argued that global communications systems do not have necessary national bases. The history of these global processes indicates that civilizations as global systems clearly predated nation-states. The basic notions of global relationships can thus be derived from the study of long-term historical trends in the macrohistorical research of the French *annales* school of historical analysis of the 1920s. "Civilizational analysis" played an important part in the eventual emergence of a cultural theory of globalization by showing that we can understand national or local historical events only in the context of world history. Unfortunately, the cultural underpinnings and consequences of these civilizational processes have often been neglected in more recent versions of the globalization thesis (Robertson 1992; Featherstone, Lash, and Robertson 1995). Indeed, the real basis for contemporary notions of the global was in cultural—or more specifically, media—processes. The idea of a global village was made popular in the media theory of Marshall McLuhan (1960), in which he contemplated the unanticipated consequences of spatial compression by the new technologies of communication. In *The Gutenberg Galaxy* (1962), McLuhan outlined the emergence of a digital age and the transformations of systems of knowledge that subsequent social philosophers, such as Jean-François Lyotard in *The Postmodern Condition* (1984), were to call postmodernization. In sociology, the first systematic definition of "globalization" was in terms of "the world as a singular system" (W. E. Moore 1966).

In general terms, globalization theory has gone through several analytical modes: nomic, cultural, and political (Axford 1995). These dimensions are currently seen as the principal components of global transformation (Held et al. 1999). In the new medical sociology, I am proposing that we need to consider a fourth stage in the theory of globalization, namely, the globalization of health risks and medical institutions. To take a specific illustration, there has been a globalization of health-measurement systems, such as DALY, under the auspices of various world health agencies. Disability is no longer conceptualized within narrow nation-state paradigms but as a global consequence of aging and chronicity. These developments in health and illness are the first steps toward a globalization of the body.

In the first phase, globalization has often been treated as

merely another stage in the growth of a world system of economic relations, the principal driving force of which has been the emergence of international and then global corporations. The economic role of global corporations within a world market is typically identified as the major cause of the partial erosion of the sovereignty of the nation-state. In turn, this erosion is identified as a condition of the failure of public policy to implement national legislation to control risk. Dissatisfaction with this emphasis on economics in world-systems theory encouraged sociologists to develop a more complex historical and causal understanding of the globalization process. Recent studies of globalization have questioned the extent of economic global integration (Hirst and Thompson 1996), while other critics have asserted the continuity of global and national economic inequality (Kalb et al. 2000).

There has been much discussion of the cultural origin and periodization of globalization processes. While globalization is a product of the late twentieth century (Giddens 1990), the existence of "world religions" prior to the advent of the modernization process is one indication that global transformation cannot be seen simply as a late consequence of modernity. Globalization is not simply a consequence of an electronic technology that made global communication possible. On the contrary, the conceptualization of the world in religious cosmology suggests distinctive and early cultural conditions for the growth of global awareness or reflexivity (Beyer 1994; Turner 1994a). Both the Greek and the Roman Empires were global systems in cultural and political terms, and they developed a tradition of cosmopolitanism, for example, in the philosophy of the Stoics.

In contemporary political movements such as antiglobalization protests, the process of globalization is often condemned
by activists as simply a modern version of Western imperial-
ism, especially as a form of American economic supremacy. The
terrorist attack on the World Trade Center gave an entirely
new significance to the idea of antiglobalization by associating
antiglobalism with Islamic anticonsumerism. Sociology has, in
any case, not only criticized the economic assumptions behind
general explanations of the global process but also rejected
the view that globalization is fundamentally Americanization
and that the hegemony of American popular culture would,
through McDonaldization (Ritzer 2000), create a standardized
and uniform global order. Anthropological contributions to the
debate quickly demonstrated that there are two consequences
of globalization that do not indicate cultural McDonaldization.
The first is the growing hybridity of cultures (Nederveen
Pieterse 1995). With migration, population transfers, open
borders, and cultural diffusion, the cultures of the urban centers of global processes become more fragmented, diversified,
and hybrid. Migration and the increase of refugees have been
critical in understanding the negative dimensions of the global
economy (Brah, Hickman, and Ghaill 1999; Sassen 1999). The
second is that, paradoxically, globalization stimulates a defense
of local cultures and traditions against incorporation into a
global system. Indeed, globalization may be in some respects a
form of translocality in which local cultures survive and are
connected by global processes. These notions gave rise eventually to the concept of glocalization, or the globalization of the
local to express the peculiar interaction between local traditions and global processes (Robertson 1992, 173–4).

For medical globalization, the issue is whether Western forms of allopathic medicine have thoroughly dominated indigenous forms of medicine. Earlier patterns of colonialism did challenge indigenous medical systems through the dominance of imperial medicine. However, homeopathic medicine in India survived British medicine and the regulation of medical professionalization, and there are important indications that global medicine involves medical pluralism. In modern Japan, for example, Western medicine is dominant because the medical schools that train doctors to practice professional medicine are situated in universities where the curriculum is taken from Western systems of medical science. After 1868, Japan adopted German medical science as the model for modernization, but Chinese medicine remains popular as a system of healing. Alongside Western medicine, one finds *kampo*, Chinese medicine that has been assimilated and transformed by Japanese ideas and customs. As a result, Japan has a mixed health system that illustrates the idea of medical pluralism.

These attempts to understand the consequences of globalization for local cultures gave rise to a political phase in the evolution of globalization theory. A debate arose over the alleged decline of the sovereignty of the nation-state (Buelens 1999). The crisis of the nation-state has raised problems about how migrants may become citizens (Aleinikoff and Klusmeyer 2000) and about the survival of citizenship rights in a context where states cannot successfully and independently enforce social rights. The decline of the state has, for some analysts, given way to the rise of the global city. New international relations involve cultural, political, and economic struggles for hegemony among global cities (A. J. Scott 2000). Urban globalism has created new risks and opportunities for cultural conflict, crime, and terrorism. The political analysis of globalization swings between extremes of pessimism in the notion of "the clash of civilizations" (Huntington 1997) and optimism in the notions of cosmopolitan democracy and virtue (Turner 1999a, 2000b). The need for some global enforcement of political rights and for the monitoring of human rights abuses has opened a sustained debate about the possibility of world government. The prospects of cosmopolitan democracy look bleak (Held 1995). The idea that the growth of human rights requires a deterritorialization of politics appears to be utopian, and the claims about the decline of the nation-state are premature (Axtman 1996). Contemporary fear of global terrorism has reinforced the political understanding of globalization by underlining the importance of the global city as a focal point of such processes. There are also political indications of the rise of transnational forms of citizenship (Bauböck 1994), and the mobility of labor, including elites, points toward the emergence of "flexible citizenship" (Ong 1999).

The human rights movement, which is particularly important for the promotion of health rights in developing societies, is a global movement that has taken root in most societies at a local level. Many local groups that are connected to each other globally by telecommunications work to improve the social and political status of women. These groups are important because, according to the economist Amartya Sen (1999), improving the education and status of women is crucial for social and economic development, and economic development is crucial to the health of the whole society. This educational-development strategy is based on the capabilities model that has been developed by the social philosopher and lawyer Martha Nussbaum (2000) with special reference to women, who often suffer most from poverty and inequality. Nussbaum points out that if women and men were treated equally—for example, if they received the same nutrition—human societies would have a surplus of women, who generally live longer than men. A ratio of more than 102 women to 100 men would be the expected sex ratio, whereas in India it is under 93 to 100. This is evidence that within the household, male children receive more nutrition. It also indicates that female infanticide is not uncommon. Local human rights groups can play an important role in protecting and supporting women in such desperate circumstances. Women often suffer from globalization in terms of the tourist sex industry and are vulnerable to infection and physical violence. Locating women's health rights in the framework of global human rights has been an important strategy in societies like the Dominican Republic, where MODEMU (Movimiento de Mujeres Unidas) has effectively lobbied the Ministry of Tourism to provide better security for women and to avoid official stigmatization of sex workers, which leads to further exploitation and discrimination (Cabezas 2002).

In mainstream sociology, globalization and risk have been understood primarily in terms of three dimensions: the economic, the cultural, and the political. There has been far less interest in the globalization of medicine and health risks, despite the ongoing HIV/AIDS epidemic. The idea of health risks has been a regular aspect of public health, epidemiology, and medical sociology for decades. For example, women with a family history of breast cancer are themselves "at risk." The importance of the idea of risk has expanded considerably in the last two decades, however, in relation to the analysis of inter-personal health risks resulting from risky sexual behavior. The HIV/AIDS epidemic produced a wealth of sociological research on the perception and management of risk in casual sexual encounters and needle etiquette among HIV-positive people. In this research, Beck's theory of risk (1992) and his and Elisabeth Beck-Gernsheim's study of modern relations of intimacy in *The Normal Chaos of Love* (1995) provided insights into risk taking and risk management. The HIV/AIDS crisis has shown yet again the close connections between the personal and the political, especially in the way relations of intimacy are bound up with the political processes of the state. The study of HIV-positive people has revealed a basic tension: love and intimacy presuppose interpersonal trust, and any sign of distrust indicates the absence of complete love. By insisting on safe sex (for example, condom use), a cautious lover shows care for his partner but may paradoxically display distrust (Rhodes and Cusick 2000). Romantic passion is threatened by questions about the partner's current health status and previous sexual practices.

Early sociological approaches to risk and HIV were dominated by practical public health concerns that concentrated on homosexual behavior. The principal issue of health education was to encourage gay men to adopt safe-sex practices. There was considerable resistance to testing for infection on grounds of civil liberties in a social environment where HIV-positive gay men were stigmatized (Patton 1990, 36). To a large extent, however, the health-education campaign in the Western world has been successful: the incidence of HIV infection was dramatically reduced in the gay community. The spread of HIV/AIDS in the heterosexual community and, specifically, the increase in female infection show that risk behavior is not exclusively confined to gay men. In the developing world, the spread of HIV to women has been an alarming development, especially because of the risk of bearing HIV-positive children. While men and women may suspect that their partners are not faithful, it is difficult for them to question a partner's behavior without undermining trust (Giffin and Lowndes 1999).

Although risk research in medical sociology has increased, there is little evidence as yet of systematic interest in the globalization of risk and its implications for individual health outcomes or national aggregate effects. In terms of the sociology of sex, Dennis Altman's recent *Global Sex* (2001) provided a unique account of the stigmatization of sexual behavior in the context of the globalization of prostitution, gay politics, AIDS, and sex tourism. Altman demonstrated that countries cannot remain totally isolated from the spread of infectious diseases and viral conditions. The social problems of AIDS education and containment gave rise to a new public health strategy that involves working with local communities and outreach groups. The new medical sociology must address a range of the conditions that are associated with globalization and risk.

RISK THEORY

How, if at all, do contemporary theories of global risk differ from the theories of their predecessors? Contemporary risk theories have three dominant features. First, they are systematic accounts that conceptualize the interaction and interdependences of the cultural, economic, and political aspects of globalization. Second, they do not embrace a uniform image of the effects of globalization. On the contrary, the consequences are seen to be contingent, uncertain, and unpredictable. Finally, they are primarily pessimistic theories of the unanticipated consequences of the global process. They are focused on the negative and unforeseen risks that our interconnected social order engenders. As we will see, there is a widely held view that the consequences of globalization for world health are generally negative. The early literature on globalization was positive, however, in that it anticipated a world of greater openness and collaboration. Theories of electronic democracy were of this order; they argued that despite the loss of local democratic participation, Web sites created new spaces for public debate, opinion formation, and political action (Vandenberg 2000). More recent political debate is skeptical about the future of democratic politics in a global world in which, ironically, communal particularity and ethnic conflict are increasing (Tourraine 2000). Globalization and its risks flow from migration, technological change, medical invention, tourism, and trade. We live in a new phase of globalization, with the spread of global health corporations and global medical markets for the diffusion of technologies, education systems, medical scientists, drugs, and organs. This phase of globalization requires a new concept because the growth of the medical economy is global. Its processes constitute "iatroglobalization," the emergence of a system of global medical exchanges through giant pharmaceutical companies, transfers of skilled medical labor, dominance by global health insurance companies, and the global sale of organs, tissues, and DNA codes. Companies associated with bioscience will be particularly influential in the evolution of iatroglobalism because they will spearhead much of the innovative technology in biotherapy—for example, cell replacement for Parkinson's disease. These bioscience companies are necessarily global, and the conditions that they aim to treat profitably are global diseases.

In *Risk Society,* Beck made a fundamental contribution to the sociology of modern society by discussing the unanticipated consequences of technology, science, and globalization for social institutions. Risk is an inevitable and necessary outcome of the process of modernization. This process gave science and technology a dominant social and economic role. Various social movements that focused on the negative effects of industrialization and modernization embraced Beck's theory. Risk society is the radicalization of modernity leading to a new stage of reflexive modernization. If primary modernization involved the rationalization of tradition, reflexive modernization means "the rationalization of rationalization" (Beck 1992, 183). Modern societies are forced to be reflexive because they are compelled to analyze and assess the complexity of the risks that challenge their existence.

Risk has changed significantly over time. Beck divided modern history into three phases: traditional society, simple modernity, and reflexive modernity. The industrialization of society involved the unequal creation of wealth, the formation of social classes, and a hierarchy of risk. Ironically, while we think of the economy as a system for the distribution of goods, risk society produces "bads." The societies of reflexive modernity involve the global distribution of bads, new patterns of status inequality, and the democratization of risks. The risks of reflexive modernity are invisible, uninsurable, systematic, generic, and democratic. While modern risks were experienced most profoundly by the working classes, the risks of reflexive modernity are democratic: we are all exposed to global warming, the hole in the ozone, and the unintended consequences of genetically modified food. Contemporary risks such as HIV/AIDS are not geographically local niche problems; they are genuinely global epidemics.

For Beck, the most useful illustration of the modernization of risk is the growth of environmental pollution and hazard. Environmental pollution is democratic because it influences all social groups regardless of their class of origin, and the risks are collective and invisible because they influence all aspects of modern life. They are not necessarily observable or palpable, however. They create a new type of community, in which solidarity is based on insecurity and anxiety rather than confidence and mutual dependence. Our anxiety about the environment creates new sets of social relations, which are structured around the individual patterns of anxiety. Risk society requires a new type of politics and brings new forms of experts into the public arena and public debate. A society based on the analysis of risk places a particular responsibility on scientists and experts in the conduct of rational debate in the public sphere. Expert opinion becomes important for shaping public debate and decision making.

The risks of contemporary society are the unintended but inevitable outcomes of the process of modernization itself, and in particular risks are products of the scientific organization of society and culture. The politicization of science, public distrust of the validity of scientific information, and lack of confidence in the neutrality of the scientific establishment are consequences of a risk society. In Europe, a number of contemporary crises associated with pollution, contaminated food, and the environment have demonstrated that governments can manipulate scientific evidence to protect their political interests. More recently, there has been extensive mistrust of government and science experts in the apparent failure to discover weapons of mass destruction in Iraq. In part, this distrust is a consequence of public misunderstanding of scientific notions of the probability of risk and acceptable levels of risk, but at a more fundamental level, risk is an inevitable outcome of rapid technological change and growing social complexity. It is the application of instrumental rationalism in the form of modern science to the production of social wealth and the management of the environment, which is itself the core of the risk society because the unintended consequences of this rationality can undermine trust and social institutions.

To this analysis of science and modernization, Beck adds the notion of reflexivity. Reflexivity is associated with the process of detraditionalization, whereby individuals and social groups become more critically aware of their own social circumstances through endless internal reflection. The idea of reflexivity therefore includes self-reflexive rational self-scrutiny and self-reflexive critical inspection. Reflexivity involves a constant critical discussion of the circumstances of modernity at both the personal and the institutional level. To some extent, risk theory follows Max Weber's understanding of rationalization as a core component of the modernization process. Rationalization involves the application of critical scientific knowledge to everyday social reality, and hence instrumental rationality corrodes traditional institutions. In an argument relating to Weber's concept of personality, risk society is associated with a new form of individualism in which the self is the product of a self-conscious process.

It is, however, somewhat misleading to place the burden of this notion of reflexivity at the individual, or subjective, level. The concept of modern risk is based on the notion that modernization brings with it a multiplication of the difficulties, problems, and contradictions that engulf modern institutions; as a result, social institutions become reflexive in the sense that the complexity of the problems they face compels them to enter into a process of collective or institutional self-evaluation and relegitimization. Modernization involves the multiplication of the contradictions within which institutions are forced to operate. The processes of problematization and contradiction are analyzed as a process of detraditionalization. Beck (1992, 153) argued that "the process of individualization is conceptualized theoretically as the product of reflexivity, in which the process of modernization as protected by the welfare state de-traditionalizes the ways of living built into industrial society."

RISK AND MEDICINE

Beck illustrated his argument with a number of examples, but his commentary on medical science is central to his general thesis (1992, 205–14). Medical practice has been protected from public scrutiny by the development of professional associations and the organization of the clinic. The clinical institution provides an organizational roof under which medical-research training and practice can be securely interrelated. It is within this professional context that medicine operates in what

Beck called an "arena of sub-politics"; that is, medicine can bypass and avoid formal political institutions to develop its own professional power base. Medicine within the experimental laboratory operates beyond the immediate scrutiny of the law and the state. Furthermore, given the speed of medical innovation and invention, the general public is typically presented with the results of the problems of medical innovation long after they are relatively well established in the experimental setting. The law and the state are often brought in to regulate medical science after the experiments and discoveries have already been achieved. The negative consequences of these developments include thalidamide babies, BSE, and CJD. These medical crises are often a consequence of inadequate health policies, poor coordination of health care, and lack of effective auditing and monitoring of services. For example, the French government has been forced to reexamine its public health policy after a series of scandals—contaminated blood, CJD, and growth hormone in the food chain. Posttransfusion blood contamination is almost eight times higher in France than in Germany. These cases indicate the importance of public health regulation in the containment of medical risk.

There is a well-established intellectual tradition of scientific dystopias that envisage science and technology as destructive to the human spirit. In modern society, these dystopian images of society have attached themselves to medical science, especially genetics (Conrad and Gabe 1999). Dystopian visions of science have been fueled by two famous accounts of the impact of science on politics: Aldous Huxley's 1932 exploration of the *Brave New World* and George Orwell's 1949 investigation of *Nineteen Eighty-Four*. Whereas Orwell's dystopia conceptualized a totalitarian regime employing information technology to control political opposition through centralized regulation, Huxley's described a humanitarian regime employing biotechnology—such as genetic manipulation, psychoactive drugs, and high-tech amusements—to accomplish social order by offering trivialized entertainment and hedonistic rewards. In the terminology of modern sociology, social order can be achieved through either medical technology or the development of a consumer culture that provides mass entertainment in parks such as Disneyland.

This dystopian tradition has been analyzed by Francis Fukuyama in *Our Posthuman Future* (2002) and by Leon Kass in *Life, Liberty, and the Defense of Dignity* (2002). Both writers endorse Huxley's biotechnological dystopia as a compelling vision of contemporary society, in which medical sciences are pushing us toward the posthumanization of the species. Both agree that the medical benefits of microbiological science are clear and potent but political interventions to establish a legal framework are necessary if we are to avoid the negative consequences of Huxley's world. According to Kass, the rational assumptions of science, advances in biotechnology, and their applications for improving health are consonant with the liberal and individualistic foundations of American democracy. Kass's argument, which in many ways replicates the assessment of science and values by Weber and Beck, is that science has the unintended consequence of eroding the social meanings that underpin fundamental social relationships. Science can help us solve practical problems, but it cannot tell us what is valuable or important. For example, applications of microbiological sciences to infertility have, through new reproductive technologies, created "extracorporeal fertilization" or "asexual reproduction" with far-reaching and unanticipated consequences for fundamental social relations, including parenthood. Reproductive technology has cut the connection between sexual intercourse and reproduction. Technology has fundamentally challenged traditional meanings of generation and parenthood. Because parenting is an important part of social citizenship, adulthood, and civic responsibility, the implications of biological technology for civil society are worrisome. In a risk society, technological advances have meant that spontaneous reproduction through heterosexual intercourse is being supplemented by planned reproduction with or without heterosexual intercourse. Lesbian parenthood has evolved through such means as adoption, surrogacy, and sperm donation, and gay parenthood is emerging through extracorporeal fertility techniques. The obvious benefits of "therapeutic cloning" for inherited disease may well pave the way for "designer babies" as a routine aspect of reproduction. For Kass and Fukuyama, the existential problem with Huxleian democracy is a paradox: while most of us will be happier and healthier, we will no longer be human.

Fukuyama is less concerned with ethical arguments about dehumanization than with the social and political implications of the new genetics. He argues that political and legal regulation is required to manage scientific innovations and their commercial exploitation. The biotechnology industry and the community of research scholars are, for obvious reasons, opposed to regulation, but Fukuyama supports regulation if it can prevent replicating past pharmaceutical catastrophes, such as sulfanilamide elixir and thalidomide, or other regulatory disasters, such as BSE and CJD. Kass supports the Bush administration on stem-cell research. Stem cells are the primordial cells that turn into the differentiated tissues that produce our vital organs, such as the liver, heart, kidney, and so forth. Stem-cell technology is a booming industry that promises to provide an endless source of replacement tissues for aging bodies. The Bush administration has taken a prudent and cautious approach that restricts the scope of such research. While Kass supports this prudent approach in the case of stem-cell research, he opposes excessive federal regulation. Prohibitions are impossible to enforce and are dangerous because the costs of interference with fundamental scientific research might be greater than the harm they actually prevent. Legislative regulation is generally ineffective and counterproductive. Kass is persuaded, therefore, that internal professional guidelines and self-regulation by scientists will be sufficient to deter the more adventurous from breaking professional norms.

There are, in general terms, three agencies or institutions that can regulate genetic research and its applications: the market, the professions, and the state. Public opinion may also exercise some degree of regulation, but it is typically expressed through the market and the state. Markets regulate institutions through the price mechanism; states achieve control by legislation; and the professions monitor their members by training, custom, and rules of conduct. Economic mechanisms, such as price regulation, are indifferent to ethical norms and may control scientific development only retrospectively. By contrast, state regulation is undermined by noncompliance, deliberate infringement, and the research opportunities that are made possible by the globalization of science. Scientists who are unhappy with the legislative constraints of their own societies may simply migrate to countries that do not exercise regulation over scientific experiment. In the United States, the National Organ Transplantation Act has attempted to impose some regulation on the internal market, but many agencies are pressing for the routine salvaging of cadaveric organs, and the American Medical Association has considered proposals to offer funeral expenses to families that donate organs. While legislation in the United States might achieve some control over the supply of organs, the globalization of the organ transplant market has been resistant to legal regulation, thereby creating intense social stratification between poor, healthy female donors from India and rich, unhealthy male recipients in the developed world (Scheper-Hughes 2001a, 2001b).

While state regulation is typically compromised by the global demand for science and professional services, professional controls are weak and ineffective. In the United Kingdom, the professional authority of the British Medical Association has been seriously undermined by a series of scandals, such as the Bristol organ crisis, which involved the unauthorized removal and storage of organs from the corpses of children who had undergone autopsies, and the report in 2003 that more than twenty thousand brains had been removed and stored without parental consent. The development of professional ethicists as advisers to regulatory boards does not appear to have achieved significant results. Many problematic developments—such as surrogate motherhood, sex selection, the appropriation of dead bodies for organ farms, and preimplantation genetic selection—have been given ethical endorsement without serious regard to deeper social or moral issues.

Globalization has made the political and legal mechanisms

available to individual states ineffective, but there are other reasons for their apparent failure. Consumer demand for healthy children, effective treatment of chronic illness, and the promise of enhanced longevity are compelling. Although many aspects of medical technology often turn out to be a "mirage of health" (Dubos 1960), consumer demands for health and longevity are not unreasonable, and hence governments are often forced by electoral pressure to satisfy them. Furthermore, in the competitive and meritorious world of science, the rewards to scientists for innovation, regardless of the social consequences, are significant. Hence, scientists who want to build reputations in growing and influential fields, such as microbiology and biotechnology, will experience strong peer pressure to compete. Corporate pressure on research agendas, especially outside the university system, is equally significant in shaping the behavior of research scientists. Salaries and promotion prospects are far greater in corporate research centers than they are in the majority of universities, especially universities that are heavily dependent on state, rather than private, funding. Scientists will, for obvious material reasons, be drawn to the corporate sector. The consequence is that their research interests and inclinations will be shaped by the need for corporate profitability.

These arguments would suggest that there is little to be done to control modern science and to protect citizens from untold medical risk. Fukuyama recognizes that regulatory controls will be difficult to enforce, but he points to the success of protests in Europe against the unregulated spread of genetically modified (GM) foods as an example of the impact of public opinion on government and market activity. As a result of environmental protests, agricultural trials of Monsanto crops in the United Kingdom have been unsuccessful, despite government support for GM crops. In response to public opinion and consumer demand, the promotion of organic food has been commercially successful as an alternative to industrialized agriculture and factory production. Nevertheless, the history of organ transplantation suggests that without international agreements and determined state regulation, local and national attempts to control biotechnology will fail in a global environment.

Regulatory controls over individual liberties are, in any case, difficult to implement in Western democracies, which champion personal freedoms. This tension between the individual and the state is particularly evident in terms of sexual activity between individuals in private. In the past, states have attempted to control sexual activity—for example, the spread of sexually transmitted diseases—and have waged educational campaigns to promote the use of condoms, but Western democratic states have been reluctant to control the spread of AIDS through the use of criminal law. The idea that governments might seek to regulate sexual practice is seen as a fulfillment of Huxley's *Brave New World.* The separation of private sex acts from reproduction by means of technology does complicate the legal issue. Do individuals have an unrestrained right to reproduce by whatever technological means possible, regardless of the implications for social identities and relationships? The social implications of this question are disturbing because we do not have clear and convincing answers. In the absence of clear social policies and values, the biotechnological advance, along with its associated risks, proceeds without effective control or direction.

Risk Society: A Critique

The model of risk society provides an insightful paradigm for the study of medical sciences and their unintended consequences, but there are four fundamental criticisms of Beck's initial theory that we should consider. First, Beck treated risk as the equivalent of hazard. His principal illustrations were Bhopal, Three Mile Island, Chernobyl, global warming, the pollution of the Black Forest, and so forth. These are perfectly good illustrations of his argument, but they should be regarded as examples of environmental and industrial hazard rather than risk. Paradoxically, Beck did not provide us with a sophisticated definition of risk, and he failed to draw on an existing tradition of research that was concerned with understanding cultural risk and blame. Mary Douglas (1992; M. Douglas and Wildavsky 1982) demonstrated the importance of recognizing cultural ambiguity and uncertainty in risk relationships rather than simply looking at tangible hazards in the environment. Beck's typology contrasted traditional and modern risks, but his approach did not allow him to distinguish systematically among hazards, risks, uncertainties, probabilities, and contingency. He was thus forced to define social or cultural risks within the paradigm of environmental hazard. In order to develop a comprehensive theory, Beck would need to distinguish more effectively between cultural risks, which are products of social complexity, and technological risks, which are effects of the breakdown of political control and regulation. His theory lacks an anthropological grasp of the cultural risks of reflexive modernity.

Second, his dichotomy exaggerated the differences between traditional and high-modern risk. The Black Death of the fourteenth century destroyed about one-third of the population of Europe and was carried by the early manifestations of global society, namely, intercontinental trade and warfare. Despite the limitations of trade routes, Greenland, too, suffered from the epidemic (McNeill 1976). The plague broke out in 1346 among the armies of a Mongol prince who was attacking the Crimea. It was democratic in that it attacked all levels of society without discrimination. While the buboes that appeared on the victims were palpable, the pathological causation was not known or fully understood. The plague became a persistent but unpredictable feature of society. In addition, it brought about a new consciousness. "Reflexive traditionalism" we might call it: a macabre sense of the ever-present reality of malevolent destruction, evil, and death. Comparisons with modern epidemics, such as malaria, and their complex social and political history are useful historically and sociologically. TB is another example of a disease that created a special consciousness, especially among an intellectual elite that included John Keats and Charlotte Brontë (Dormandy 1999). The globalization of disease was powerfully illustrated in 1918, with the outbreak of the Spanish influenza pandemic, which killed twenty-five million people in six months—about three times the number of deaths in the First World War. An epidemic of encephalitis lethargica and a further outbreak of influenza followed in 1920. These epidemics were rapid and global because the war had brought about massive movements of people. Influenza spread rapidly among American soldiers. Between September and October 1918, 20 percent of the American army was ill and twenty-four thousand soldiers died of flu, compared with thirty-four thousand in battle. From these examples, it is evident that no clear point in history divides simple from reflexive modernity, and popular images or metaphors of AIDS are not far removed from the baroque vision of death (Turner 1994a; Ziegler 1998).

Third, Beck's theory was weak in its attribution of political responsibility for the risky nature of society. Are risks the inevitable outcome of the sheer complexity and diversity of technology in high modernity? Are there significant differences in terms of political culpability for certain crises? Recent reports on the origins of the BSE crisis suggest that the British government's management was faulty and secretive. Similarly, was the outbreak of HIV/AIDS the unfortunate and contingent consequence of hunting and eating monkeys or the consequence of oral polio vaccine that was contaminated by diseased cells from chimpanzee kidneys? The risks associated with the global spread of drugs also reflect government policies and legislation regulating drug use. We need to distinguish, then, between voluntary risk, in which governments accept the presence of risk as an unavoidable aspect of social change (such as car accidents), and involuntary risk, in which a risk is imported without the knowledge or consent of a government (for example, acid rain or global warming or SARS). Thus, "traded risks" cross national borders as a consequence of economic exchange while "public risks" are the opposite of a "public good."

Fourth, Beck's theory has so far failed to connect systematically the growth of the institutions of social citizenship and human rights with the globalization of risk. Beck's view of global risk in the 1990s did not include any notion of global terrorism, nor did it consider the complex relationship between civil liberties, global terror, and political risk. The development of human rights legislation and global surveillance are in some measure consequences of risk society. While risk theory has concentrated on the distribution of "bads," a positive but unintended consequence of global risk is the emergence of a global consensus at the governmental level that human beings have a right to a safe environment. This set of human rights has evolved for two basic reasons. First, problems of the global order, such as the spread of AIDS or the pollution of the environment, cannot be solved by the unilateral action of individual governments. Second, the social risks that are created by new technologies such as cloning and GM food do not easily fit into the existing politico-legal framework. The growth of involuntary risk for individual societies is the context of the growth of global responses in terms of a new regime of rights and regulations.

Is Beck's theory worth saving? The criticisms are intended to extend rather than destroy his account of risk. There are two obvious ways in which his approach can be further elaborated. That is, we need to distinguish more clearly between types of risks. The cultural dimension of medical risks is a critical aspect of political responses—for example, to the stigmatization of HIV/AIDS sufferers. And we need to have a better understanding of the voluntary and involuntary aspects of risks that governments face in a global context. Global warming may be an involuntary hazard of modern forms of transportation. Lung cancer may be an avoidable risk of cigarette smoking, which can be regulated by government legislation—for example, by banning tobacco advertising or increasing taxes on cigarettes. Beck's criticisms of the negative consequences of modernization and globalization are important, but his theory does not involve naive pessimism about the future. His vision is not dystopian because he believes that the most effective response to the risks of social modernization is to deepen the democratic culture of society.

FROM ENVIRONMENTAL TO MEDICAL CITIZENSHIP

Concern with the negative consequences of industrial capitalism for the natural environment has become a dominant issue of global politics. Individual governments have, at various levels of intervention, attempted to protect their national populations from the effects of public and involuntary risks (acid rain, radioactive waste, and oil spills). They have also been concerned with the unpredictable consequences of the industrialization of agricultural production, carbon dioxide emissions from motor vehicles, and contamination from civil nuclear power. Howard Newby (1996), writing about the development of environmentalism in Britain, identified four stages in the emergence of "environmental citizenship." First, from 1880 to 1900, there was a concern for preservation, as epitomized by the National Trust. Second, in the interwar years, there was growing middle-class criticism of laissez faire economics and an emphasis on the need for regulation and the provision of public amenities. From the early 1960s through the 1970s, environmental anxieties were expressed in a third stage, through organizations such as Friends of the Earth and the Ecology Party. Finally, in the late 1990s, the parochial British debate

was challenged by a political recognition of the universal dimensions of global warming. With a new emphasis on sustain-
ability, the traditional language of amenity was replaced by a
discourse on global crisis and catastrophe.

A similar pattern also appeared in the growth of the U.S.
environmental lobby, where a legal framework was created to
regulate industry and protect the environment through the
Clean Air Act (1963), the Land and Water Conservation Funds
Act (1965), the Water Quality Act (1965), and the Clean Water Restoration Act (1966). After the so-called Conservation
Congress of 1968, there followed a suite of regulatory provisions: the National Environmental Policy Act, the Toxic Sub-
stances Control Act, the Occupational Safety and Health Act,
and a number of food and drug acts. Beck's concept of risk captures the critical dimension of ecological consciousness as a lack
of confidence in expert opinion and as lack of trust in government policy. There have been major public debates exposing
internal divisions in the academic community and inconsisten-
cies in the scientific evidence. The first case of BSE in Japan, in
September 2001, confirmed the global interconnectedness of
food production and distribution, where there are no closed
borders for goods or diseases. The result was an immediate decline in meat imports, which in turn had a direct impact on the
Australian economy. Against a background of distrust of government reports and expert advice, green politics gives public
expression to ecological concerns in terms of the right to a safe
and, if possible, "natural" environment.

Whereas social rights were historically the consequence of
class-based activity such as industrial strikes, contemporary human rights are frequently the result of social or environmental

movements and consumer lobbies that have diverse social memberships. Global social movements, rather than social-class conflicts, appear to be relatively successful in bringing about an expansion of rights. In the case of Taiwan, the causal connection between awareness of rights and the growth of participatory democracy is illustrated by the anti–nuclear power movement in the 1980s. Whereas national citizenship rights attempt to protect individuals from the vagaries of the marketplace, the new regime of global rights attempts to protect humans from the negative health and safety consequences of economic growth and technology. The human rights legislative framework is meant to protect future generations from the contemporary consequences of environmental degradation; ecological citizenship embraces the notion of justice as a generational issue.

While the environmental lobby and the emergence of green, or ecological, citizenship were shaped by a sociological concern with the impact of industrial capitalism on the environment, the second dimension of this debate involved an anthropological awareness of the impact of capitalism and colonial powers not only on the environment but also on human communities. If unrestrained industrial capitalism had negative effects on the natural environment, then the obvious conclusion is that the spread of capitalist agriculture has devastating consequences for traditional societies. The destruction of "primitive society" was not simply a consequence of military encounters or the ravages of European disease; it also involved the removal of aboriginal societies from their land in order to create a global market in beef, sheep, and cereals. In the United States, the end of the Civil War, in 1865, created the conditions for the commercial exploitation and settlement of the West. The destruction of indigenous nomadic cultures was an effect of the destruction of the buffalo, which occurred in order to exploit the plains for beef production. The Great Sioux War ended tragically at Wounded Knee in December 1890. The American frontier, so important for the evolution of American individualism, began to close. In the 1870s and again in the 1890s, Native Americans adopted new dancing ceremonies that expressed the hope that deceased ancestors and diminished food sources would return to earth and restore communities facing extermination. These new ceremonies, later called the Ghost Dance movement, are an illustration of traditional reflexivity, in which the destruction of the Plains culture gave rise to charismatic movements that carried a new mentality (Niezen 2000). In the nineteenth century, the spread of capitalist agriculture, the destruction of aboriginal cultures, and white migration created the characteristics of white-settler society from the American Northwest to South Island, New Zealand. In the twentieth century, these societies have experienced a common pattern of policy making designed to acculturate, assimilate, or accommodate aboriginal peoples. This pattern of global development raises serious questions about the allegedly democratic nature of the risks of reflexive modernity.

We can conceptualize a range of rights relating to the environment, aboriginal entitlements to land, and cultural rights of identity that are closely connected with the globalization process. Understanding the relationship between the exploitation of land and the destruction of aboriginal cultures has given rise to a more comprehensive debate about cultural rights in a global society. Whereas the national framework of citizenship had little analytical light to shed on the problem of ethnic identity, the global aboriginal issue spurred more fundamental discussions relating to identity and difference. The third type of citizenship rights thus involves culture. Cultural rights to language, to a share in the cultural heritage of a community, to freedom of religion and belief, and ultimately to identity have become central to contemporary politics, but these cultural rights have neither precise nor necessary connections to membership in the nation-state. They depend on international covenants.

These emerging rights (to a safe environment, to aboriginal culture and land, and to ethnic identity) point to and are underpinned by a generic right, to ontological security as a parallel to social security. This right is the foundation for a new medical citizenship that broadly encompasses the right to health. Human beings are characterized by their frailty and vulnerability and by the precarious character of their social and political arrangements (Turner 2000c, 2001a). Citizenship is a sociopolitical system that provides some protection from the particular risks of an advanced society. Where life is nasty, brutish, and short, citizenship functions to make the world more secure and civilized. The irony of globalization is that in many respects our world is becoming more risky and more precarious because the dangers of modern technology often outweigh, or at least cast doubt on, its advantages.

The basic right of ontological security is closely connected to questions of human embodiment, but it goes beyond reproductive rights and involves entitlement to respect. The right to ontological security underpins other environmental, cultural, and identity claims characteristic of modern social movements.

In this context, medical citizenship can be deployed as a collective umbrella for this cluster of rights. Ontological security can be safeguarded only by a set of values that promote stewardship of the environment, concern for precarious human communities, recognition of cultural differences, and respect for human dignity. In short, we need a set of obligations that correspond to the demand for human rights. These rights to ontological security are closely tied to recognition of women's rights and to the risks of unregulated economic development.

These three postnational components of citizenship rights (ecological, aboriginal, and cultural) are identified here as analogous to the three stages of the historical development of national citizenship (Marshall 1963). They form a hierarchy: environment, community, and human beings. These new rights are conceptually and historically connected by the risks to human embodiment in a global system. Postnational environmental rights are connected by human frailty and by the fact that the nation-state cannot adequately respond to this vulnerability within an ecological system that is globally disrupted by modern technology. What is less clear is the presence of an institutional structure to which these rights correspond. National citizenship rights were matched by the rise of specific institutional structures: courts of justice, parliamentary institutions, and the welfare state. Environmental, aboriginal, and cultural rights are all enshrined in components of the Universal Declaration of Human Rights and, more recently, in the legal recommendations arising from U.N. conferences on the environment (Rio de Janeiro), population (Cairo), and human settlements (Istanbul), but as yet there is no decisive set of global governmental arrangements that enforce or match these rights.

The notion that there should be global governance has been canvassed by numerous social scientists, but we still need to spell out how a global political community could exist and exercise legitimate power.

REGULATION AND RISK

In contemporary sociology, two publications profoundly influenced the sociological imagination about modern capitalism: Ulrich Beck's *Risk Society* (1992) and George Ritzer's *McDonaldization of Society* (2000). Yet they carried profoundly different interpretations of our modern condition. For Beck, late capitalism is contingent, unstable, risky, and uncertain, whereas Ritzer argued that society is becoming homogenized and predictable. The processes and systems of standardization mean that McSociety lacks surprises (Turner 1999a). While these two accounts of high modernity appear to be totally contradictory, the two processes are related by a systematic dialectic. We can imagine a sequence in which the growth of risks eventually results in a systemic crisis or indeed a major catastrophe that produces the need for greater regulation. Governments typically react to such crises by creating a system of regulatory controls, which characteristically employ auditing of risks and develop risk registers. Audits are therefore as important as risks. In an advanced industrial society, regulatory control systems tend to produce a political reaction that calls for the return of the free market, the reduction of state intervention, a return to liberal values, and the restoration of individual freedoms. There is a perpetual cycle of regulation and deregulation whereby governments that promote deregulation bring about a return to a risk environment.

These cycles of regulation and deregulation shape the history of successive governments in Western societies. The pattern of American politics can be described as an endless oscillation of regimes of regulation and deregulation (Eisner 1993). The Great Depression and the Second World War required state intervention on a massive scale and extensive legislation to mobilize society. In a similar fashion, the New Deal produced a considerable volume of legislation to protect workers from the social risks of unemployment and the hazards of industrial technology. These regulatory regimes were followed by deregulation of the economy and technological systems. In particular, economic stagflation produced an "efficiency regime" that attempted to liberate the market and production from state controls. A similar pattern of policies shaped British political history, where the regulatory legacy of social Keynesianism was finally destroyed by the neoconservative policies of Margaret Thatcher's and John Major's governments.

Globalization has intensified the dialectic of risk and regulation because few governments can successfully regulate their own economies in a context of global competition. Global corporations simply transfer their operations to locations where government or union intervention is minimal. Crime works on the same principle. Globalization has simply expanded the opportunities for Mafia-like organizations to proliferate, especially in the global drug market. Organized crime, like consumerism generally, is now an important feature of the emerging globalized culture (Findlay 2000). In Southeast Asia and in Africa, the global drug barons are an inescapable component of the state. Such globalized drug systems threaten world health through drug dependency, commercialized sex, and the exploitation of child sex workers. Attempts by nation-states to control the drug trade are highly selective in their levels of permission and prohibition. The history of the regulation of tobacco is a classic example and illustrates the dialectical pattern of risk, audit, regulation, and deregulation. The growth of globalization creates both an environment of risk and a set of opportunities for the expansion of social rights. Without an expansion of citizenship, the globalization of risk will have wholly negative consequences for health and well-being. In conclusion, we can see the expansion of social citizenship on a national basis and the growth of human rights protection on a global level in terms of a new sociolegal phenomenon that we may simply call medical citizenship.

CONCLUSION: MEDICAL CITIZENSHIP

In *The History of Sexuality* (1979), Foucault distinguished between the regulation of the individual body and the regulation of populations. In the same vein, we can think about citizenship as providing legal solutions for the management of individuals and populations. Social citizenship has expanded with the rise of modern administration through the nation-state. It is an aspect of the modernization of societies in which the state takes responsibility for developing the potential of individuals and populations by means of health policies. These health interventions are often benign, such as dietary instructions to pregnant women or the encouragement of Boy Scout organizations to improve the fitness of the male population. With the development of National Socialism, these processes of health modernization took on a more dangerous and sinister direction through state eugenics programs.

As a result of global changes, we are moving toward a new medical citizenship that will increasingly be expressed through human rights legislation. The global foundations of medical citizenship were established by the Universal Declaration of Human Rights in 1948, in Article 25, which says that "[e]veryone has the right to a standard of living adequate for the health and well-being of himself and his family, including food, clothing, housing and medical care and necessary social services." WHO adopted a global strategy, "Health for All by the Year 2000," that attempted to address the health divide between rich and poor societies. A major concern of WHO has been the provision of global support for malaria-control programs. Malaria is endemic in many African societies, and there are annually more than two million deaths from malaria in Africa. The global attempts to eradicate diseases such as polio, TB, and malaria are contributions to medical rights. In many cases, it is difficult to detach medical citizenship from reproductive citizenship since health for women is closely bound up with women's right to reproduce under conditions of their own choosing. Furthermore, the right to health cannot be detached from more general questions of social equality and security. Lack of educational opportunity for women is an essential feature of their poor health and their inability to secure their reproductive rights. Health is an outcome of a complex web of rights that attempt to address issues of justice in a world where such questions can find only global solutions.

Chapter Eight
THE NEW MEDICAL SOCIOLOGY

INTRODUCTION: GLOBALIZATION AND CORPORATE POWER

ALTHOUGH CONVENTIONAL MEDICAL SOCIOLOGY involves the study of health and illness in specific societies (Cockerham 2001), a central claim of this book is that globalization has changed the context within which we can study health and illness. The HIV/AIDS epidemic is a useful illustration of the developments that have accompanied globalization. AIDS is both a consequence and a cause of globalization because it spreads through global interconnectedness and increases global consciousness. It requires a global medical and economic response. By 1979, awareness of HIV/AIDS and ARC quickly changed governments' complacent attitude toward the epidemic. In the West, the HIV/AIDS epidemic was a warning that the era of acute infectious disease was not over. While travel has played an important role in the development of AIDS, the origins of HIV/AIDS are controversial. Tourism, trade, and migration have spread HIV/AIDS, and it is a major example of how globalization has increased the presence of infectious disease. Increases in TB are also an effect of HIV infection. Thus, globalization has integrated world health into a single, highly interconnected system. Whereas diseases in the past existed in specialized geographic niches, the interconnectedness of the global economy has meant the interconnectedness of disease, or at least the risk of disease (McNeill 1976). By the mid-1990s, ninety-seven million people traveled by air between the United States and other societies. The spread of SARS in 2003 demonstrated the dangers of political secrecy and forced the Chinese authorities to adopt an open and cooperative relationship with WHO and the Association of South East Asian Nations. Pessimistic epidemiologists sound increasingly like neo-Malthusians because of the return of "old" conditions, such as outbreaks of TB in the developed world and the global spread of more exotic conditions—Marburg virus, Ebola, and Lassa fever. These outbreaks have drawn attention to the continuity of infectious disease in the developed world—one-third of deaths in the United States in the 1990s were from infectious disease. Contemporary risks such as HIV/AIDS and SARS are not local, niche problems; they are genuinely global epidemics and harbingers of a global consciousness.

This study is based on the view that conventional medical sociology has made major contributions to knowledge but it does not fully grasp key aspects of global modernity. We need a greater emphasis on economics, politics, rights, and citizenship in order to provide a more comprehensive and sophisticated understanding of health and illness in the contemporary world. The new medical economy requires a new medical sociology. The concept of a medical economy recognizes that the major economic processes of a modern society are concerned with the production of health through the pharmaceutical industry, research and development in genetics, the integration of microbiology and information science, and the management of life processes, such as reproduction, aging, and death. Medicine as a social institution is a major component of this global economy. In more direct terms, the medical economy is based on the production, reproduction, and management of the human body. Historically, the word *economy* referred to the management of the resources of a household, and a medical economy is thus the management of the body as a resource of a society. An economy is, in general, concerned with the management of scarcity. A medical economy is the effective organization of the genetic resources of a community with the aim of maximizing and rationalizing those scarce resources. The task of medical sociology is to understand and to explain the social processes that underpin this new economy. The global health economy requires a new sociological paradigm—the new medical sociology.

THE MODERN CONTEXT OF MEDICINE

Eliot Freidson, in *Profession of Medicine* (1970), proposed that the success of the medical profession rested not only on its political power but also on the trust of the public. These two dimensions of professionalism are medical dominance and the consulting ethic. Medical dominance requires the support of the state, and the consulting ethic depends on public confidence and trust. These dimensions have been transformed by the growth of corporate and global medical systems. This corporate development of the commercial potential of health and illness marks the emergence of the global medical economy. These global changes are destroying the traditional doctor-patient relationship, but they are also opening up possibilities, the future directions of which remain unclear.

In terms of the growth of public confidence and trust in the medical profession, a variety of technical inventions and discoveries of nineteenth-century medicine, such as immunization, established the scientific authority of medicine as a profession. In Britain in 1858, the Medical Register excluded practitioners of traditional medicine, such as herbalists and bonesetters (R. Porter 2001). For the lay public, improvements in survival rates from surgery have been especially visible evidence of the scientific basis of contemporary medical practice. The effectiveness of twentieth-century surgery was consolidated through improvements in anaesthesia, electrolyte physiology, and cardiopulmonary physiology. The use of "keyhole surgery" has also provided palpable evidence of medical improvements. Although the quality of general practice still depends in large measure on interpersonal skills that can be fully acquired only through experience rather than formal training, the status of medical institutions in society depends significantly on "hard" science and technology. Medical technology promises significant therapeutic improvement in the management of health and illness, but it also brings significant risks to well-being, individual rights, and social stability. The storage of genetic information about individuals for policing, forensic investigations, actuarial calculations of insurance risk, employment inquiries, and general surveillance poses significant problems for individual liberties. New reproductive technologies have the potential to transform family life and kinship relations.

In order to gain the full benefit of medical innovation, there will have to be some regulation of the social and cultural risks associated with cloning, new reproductive technologies, organ transplants, and genetic screening. Who should exercise these regulatory constraints in order to achieve governance over medical science? Neither the professions nor governments are able to deliver effective oversight because the globalization of markets makes legislative and political regulation problematic. The result is an endless cycle of risk, audit, regulation, and deregulation. The cycle further inflames lay suspicion of expert opinion and erodes the relationship of trust between patients and doctors. In Britain, a number of major scandals and crises in the health system have tested the limits of the legal framework of medicine. The British Medical Association has been attacked for its failure to monitor effectively doctors who have been charged with criminal offenses or malpractice. Shortages of doctors and nurses in the NHS have reinforced the general sense of crisis and poor management. The emergency recruitment of nurses from India only underlined a general crisis in recruitment in the British health system. The apparent contradictions in the expert advice relating to the British foot-and-mouth epidemic of 2001 further illustrated the problematic authority of scientific or expert opinion. Volatile feelings of trust and distrust in expert systems have become a major issue of modern society. Sociology could help us understand this problem by reexamining technology, risk, and opportunity and by considering whether international agreements or a global framework is feasible in managing the medical economy.

Any understanding of medicine in contemporary society will have to examine the economics of the corporate structure of medical practice and locate that corporate structure within a set of global processes. This study has already drawn attention to the risks associated with the globalization of disease and the new pandemics. These sociological debates about risk, globalization, and technology may often appear overly abstract, but they have in fact a direct relevance to policy and research issues relating to new medical technologies. Globalization has played a major role in the spread of new infectious diseases since the 1980s, such as HIV/AIDS, hepatitis, and the Ebola virus. Hollywood films—*Plague, Outbreak,* and *Congo*—have given popular expression to the public fear of the new plagues (Petersen and Lupton 1996). There has also been the spread of the "old" infectious diseases (TB, malaria, typhoid, and cholera). These diseases have had significant negative consequences for the economies of the developing world, but they will also reappear in the affluent West as a consequence of the globalization of transportation, tourism, and labor markets. The deregulation of global markets by the neoconservative policies of Reagan and Thatcher had the unintended consequence of enhancing the globalization of disease. It is unlikely that corporations will adopt policies of corporate citizenship quickly enough to exercise restraint and institutionalize environmental audits to regulate their impact on local communities. These global developments have also created new opportunities for the exercise of consumer power as a challenge to the negative impact of corporate enterprise on fragile communities and environments.

Future research into health must be connected to existing debates about civil society and citizenship (Alexander 1994). Citizenship entitlements to health would include reproductive rights, but they would also embrace rights to a clean environment, adequate food and water supplies, and appropriate medical services. We need to realize more clearly that health is a fundamental entitlement of social citizenship, alongside education and welfare. Health entitlements are often difficult to implement within a world economy in which risks are global. Health as entitlement raises difficult political and policy questions because there is an inevitable tension between social citizenship as a national system of rights and obligations and human rights as a system of entitlements separate from the sovereignty of particular nation-states.

Globalization, the commercialization of medical care, and the creation of free markets in body parts have also had important consequences for the professional model of health care. The model of the professional doctor that shaped Talcott Parsons's approach to the professions and values in the 1950s is now obsolete, with the passing of the "golden age of doctoring." In American medical sociology, the publication of Paul Starr's *Social Transformation of American Medicine* (1982) was a major indication of the changing relationship between the physician, the patient, the corporation, and the state. We have already seen that between 1875 and 1920 the status of the general practitioner in the United States was transformed by a number of social developments. The expansion in the market for medical services in this period was a consequence of economic growth, urbanization, and the development of urban transportation systems. The sovereignty and autonomy of the medical profession were reinforced by the development of licensing laws with state backing. With the professional development of medicine, physicians came to oppose forms of medical practice that departed from the fee-for-service model. Alternative medicine went into retreat. The professional associations of medicine were generally critical of any political control of health that was seen to be a threat to professional autonomy. The professions claimed that collectivist innovations in the delivery of health care would undermine the principles of individualism, self-help, and self-reliance on which American health care had been built. In addition, the development of diagnostic and preventive medicine by public health departments would have been a direct economic threat to the medical profession and would have challenged its professional autonomy and its control over the relationship with the patient.

Welfare and health programs in the United States did not develop in the same direction as they had in Europe, partly because socialist politics, welfare traditions, and working-class movements were relatively weak. The major divisions in American society were thought to be ethnic or related to social status rather than economic class. There was no significant working-class challenge to the existing capitalist economic and social system, which championed individualism, community responsibility, and associational politics. Historically, the American system has depended far more on philanthropic support, voluntary associations, and private insurance than on centralized state provision. The American political tradition interprets entitlement in terms of a rights-conscious citizen model, not in terms of welfare institutions (Schudson 1998). Although there was a significant expansion of welfare provision as a result of the Social Security Act of 1935, the New Deal, and civil rights agitation, as late as 1967 the participation rate for those who were eligible for welfare was only 42 percent. There was relatively little continuous and effective political agitation for state-welfare systems such as compulsory health insurance. In the mid-1930s Depression era, however, the American Medical Association eventually accepted the view that some features of private insurance could support its monopoly on medical care.

By securing the maximum provider control, the professional association was able to convert third-party insurance to its financial advantage. In the postwar period, the organized medical profession was also able to secure significant political and financial advantages from the development of Medicaid, Medicare, and other medical programs.

The modern development of corporate control over medical care has contributed to the decline of professional autonomy, initiative, and social status. The free market and aggressive entrepreneurship have brought about a decline in the social status of general practitioners by converting them to the hired employees of profit-making, private-sector health corporations. The professional physician hired by a commercial enterprise has to make a profit in addition to providing an adequate system of health care. Furthermore, the contemporary development of health care in the United States has brought about a new emphasis on medical specialization, which has undermined the occupational coherence and solidarity of medicine as a professional group. In addition to this internal division, the growth of consumer groups, malpractice legislation, and public alarm in response to technological medicine have created a renewed interest in more holistic, alternative, and complementary systems. The commercialization of medicine and the dominance of free-market principles have eroded the foundations of the traditional autonomous professional physician as an individual provider of care in a direct relationship with the client.

While free-market policies may have changed the conditions under which the traditional autonomy of the medical profession was sustained, they have also had serious consequences for users and consumers, which have become apparent in a variety of areas of welfare. For example, U.S. poverty has increased by 30 percent among children since 1979. In the early 1980s, the infant mortality rate increased in eleven states. Considerable differences between black and white mortality rates have persisted. In Michigan, infant mortality rates rose for the first time in more than thirty years to more than thirteen per one thousand live births. The increase in the infant mortality rate is associated with the increase in poverty and unemployment, a decline in nutrition, and the loss of health insurance coverage through new limits on Medicaid. The health-care crisis was manifest in the rising number of uninsured Americans, increasing use of CAM, increasing health inequalities, and the growth of self-help movements (McKinlay and Stoeckle 1988).

While there are significant indicators of increasing poverty, the private health sector has enjoyed buoyant profits and expansion. The economic and political importance of the Reagan tax cuts was that by reducing revenue to the state, they curtailed the government's ability to introduce new social welfare programs that would have removed hardship, stimulated employment, and restored welfare measures. Their consequences in public provision have reinforced the class divisions within the health-care system, resulting in a marked division between the privileged and the poor. In Britain, similar changes have exacerbated conflicts between private practice and the NHS and have virtually removed services such as dentistry from collective provision. As medicine has become increasingly specialized, the general practitioner has become the conduit who refers patients to specialists further along on the chain of delivery. The continuity of care and the trust in the family doctor that characterized traditional medical practice have been eroded by the commercialization of services and the increasing anonymity of medical practitioners in relation to patients.

Sociologists have attempted to understand these developments within the framework of global risk. Of course, anxiety about the pace of technology and its unintended—and often pernicious—consequences has been a feature of public inquiry into medicine for a considerable time. In the postwar period, doctors, especially in research hospitals, were criticized for their fascination with medical technology, and it was feared that technological developments would undermine traditional patient-centered care (Wolf and Berle 1981). Scientific anxieties about medical harm and public concern about adverse drug reactions began to appear in the medical literature in the 1950s and 1960s. With the expansion of the legal rights of patients, trust between patients and their doctors has been tested by the emergence of an aggressive culture of litigation. Medical malpractice suits have become an important part of modern legal practice, and lack of confidence in medical practice has become a contentious arena in public life. There has been an erosion of public confidence in the medical profession. At the same time, the technological problems of medicine have become global, and the risks of medical failure or mismanagement have enormous legal and economic consequences for the health-care system. The often-spectacular growth of medical sciences has presented new opportunities and corresponding risks for medical practice.

The development of new reproductive technologies, genetic engineering, and the enhancement of human traits are part of a second medical revolution, one that combines microbiology,

computerization, and information science (Foss and Rothenberg 1987). This revolution is a threat to traditional institutions and religious cosmologies, but it may also challenge the
processes of political governance. The modern notion of risk
society critically evaluates the unintended consequences of
medical change, the question of whether the technological imperative can be regulated, and the relationship between pure
research, commercialization, and academic autonomy. For example, pharmaceutical companies have turned to contract research organizations rather than universities to undertake basic
research on drugs. In the United States, about 60 percent of
industry-based pharmaceutical grants have gone to contract research outside the traditional universities. These commercial
organizations are economically efficient, but they are also less
independent and less critical than academic institutions. The
scientific community has argued that commercial research is
not systematically published and unlikely to be critical of pharmaceutical products. Private modes of research are not compatible with the public norms of publication, debate, and
criticism that are essential to scientific objectivity. The fact
that the pharmaceutical industry is currently dominated by a
limited number of corporations poses serious problems for the
regulation of the industry and market freedom.

One significant illustration of the controversial and complex
relationships between corporate enterprise and the public university can be taken from the signing of the "Novartis-Berkeley
Strategic Alliance" in November 1998. The Swiss pharmaceutical and agrochemical company Novartis agreed to pay the
Department of Plant and Microbial Biology of the University
of California's Berkeley campus twenty-five million dollars in

research support over five years. This alliance has often been
disturbed by changes in the global economy of agbiotech—for
example, by lack of economic confidence in the industry—but
the alliance has also been questioned by leading academics at
Berkeley. On the positive side, some Berkeley professors have
argued that the cash injection has had beneficial effects on the
quantity and the quality of research undertaken in the department. Critics of the alliance have argued that the presence of
Novartis precluded the development of alternative research
strategies, technologies, and educational programs. The secretive nature of the design and implementation of the agreement
disrupted collegial relationships within the faculty. The alliance did not give rise to lively and critical interdisciplinary
research teams, and the experimental nature of the initiative
was not properly measured or monitored. These difficulties
pinpoint more general problems in attempts to integrate private business into public institutions at a national level, but
there are also global difficulties.

There has been considerable international disagreement and
conflict over the most appropriate strategies for combating the
spread of AIDS, especially in Africa. Some politicians favor investing in preventive and educational strategies to warn young
people of the dangers of unprotected sex. Alternatively, some
political leaders take the view that priority should be given to
treating the victims of AIDS with appropriate drugs. The
problem is that the legal patents on drugs often make them
unaffordable. These policy conflicts were the political background to the Doha agreement of November 2001, which recognized the right of countries to override the drug patents of
major corporations in order to provide affordable health care,

and it compiled a list of appropriate diseases to which monopolistic patent rights would not apply, such as AIDS, TB, malaria, and a range of tropical ailments. Cancer, asthma, and diabetes were not included in the agreement. The pharmaceutical companies were under pressure to reach an international agreement at Doha because they had come under considerable public relations criticism following protests by HIV-positive South Africans. In South Africa, 20 percent of pregnant women are infected with HIV, and 80 percent of AIDS-related deaths are in sub-Saharan Africa. The South African Treatment Action Campaign claims that there are 4.7 million sufferers and six hundred deaths per day. Following the anthrax attacks in the United States, the U.S. and Canadian governments wanted to ensure adequate supplies of Cipro to treat strains of the anthrax disease and so threatened to overturn Bayer's patent on the drug. These events in South Africa and the United States put the pharmaceutical companies on the defensive, and the Doha agreement was welcomed as a major step toward reducing the cost of treatment for major diseases in developing societies.

However, the Doha agreement was seen to be a commercial threat to intellectual property rights and the profitability of patents, and the agreement's provisions have consequently been steadily compromised by restrictions on its scope. These compromises include restricting the countries that can override patents, limiting the qualifying technologies, and creating complex and expensive legal provisions. Both the U.S. trade representative and the European Union trade commissioner have sought to limit the number of diseases covered by the original agreement. The failure to reach a viable agreement

demonstrates the economic influence of the global pharmaceutical corporations over governments and their ability to thwart
WHO objectives promoting egalitarian health conditions
(Love 2003). Corporate patent rights have prevented a satisfactory solution to a problem that is threatening the whole of
Africa. The problem of intellectual property rights demonstrates the broader issues of global regulation of markets in relation to the delivery of essential health services.

REGULATION, THE PROFESSIONS, AND SCIENTIFIC KNOWLEDGE

Regulation and deregulation are characteristic policy cycles
that follow successive governments in the United States and
the United Kingdom. The American Great Depression and the
Second World War required extensive state intervention and
comprehensive legislation to mobilize society behind the war
effort, just as the New Deal produced legislation to protect
workers from unemployment and the hazards of industrial
technology, but subsequent laissez faire regimes deregulated
the economy and technological systems (Eisner 1993). The end
of the Clinton presidency and the election of President George
W. Bush have provided another reversal in the dialectic between regulation and deregulation. Clinton's raft of regulatory
devices has been negated by the Bush administration's rejection
of the Kyoto Protocol and other environmental measures. A
similar pattern shaped recent British political history, with the
Thatcher and Major governments finally abandoning the legacy
of social Keynesianism.

Globalization has intensified the dynamic relationship of
risk and regulation. In the contemporary political environment, few governments can successfully regulate their own

economies in a context of global competition. The attempt by governments to both promote and regulate research with respect to human genetics is perhaps the most dramatic illustration of the dynamic between regulation and risk. In 2001, President Bush, responding to pressure from religious groups, attempted to regulate genetic research by confining state-funded programs to a limited number of stem-cell lines. This regulation has forced some university research groups to secure supplies of stem cells from fertility clinics for privately financed research. The U.S. National Institutes of Health has expressed concern that there may be supply problems for federally funded research with many of the sixty-four stem lines that have been recognized by the president's ruling. In addition, legal conflicts over ownership of genetics patents may make supply from privately funded institutes problematic. Governance and regulation are difficult in the case of genetics research.

With the triumph of the neoconservative economic strategy of deregulation and privatization beginning in the early 1980s, the problems of global regulation have intensified. Deregulation and competition in the global pharmaceutical industries have caused profound crises. The growth of litigation in class-action suits against drug companies is an important illustration of the contradictions of free markets and regulatory devices. It is widely acknowledged that all medical treatments have some side effects, but the drug corporations have been protected from litigation because their products were licensed by government agencies like the U.S. Food and Drug Administration (FDA). In addition, many drugs are not sold directly to customers because doctors are responsible for prescriptions. One consequence of the HIV/AIDS epidemic of the 1980s was the

FDA's decision to accelerate the approval of drugs, but an unintended consequence of that aspect of deregulation was an increase in the negative side effects of drugs, especially in the case of irritable bowel disorders and diabetes.

In the quest for higher profits, pharmaceutical companies are directing their advertisements directly to the customer rather than to the traditional intermediary, the doctor. For instance, antidepressant drugs were originally welcomed as safe alternatives to tricyclic antidepressants because deliberately overdosing on those drugs is virtually impossible. As a result, Prozac emerged as a major lifestyle drug. Another drug, Paxil, was the subject of a lawsuit in which a jury decided that it was largely responsible for the murder of a family by a man taking the drug as an antidepressant. The compensation in such cases of product litigation in the United Sates will not seriously undermine the market, but it does indicate the complex relationships between regulation and deregulation.

Controlling the specific risks of medical practice and medical sciences has proved particularly difficult. Both the medical profession and the government have been found wanting in the contemporary regulatory context. In the 1950s, the theory of professionalization was a dominant concern of sociologists because the professions and professional culture held the promise of some degree of normative regulation and the imposition of standards of service that would counteract the naked exuberance and destructiveness of the capitalist market. The theory contrasted forms of regulation of the doctor-patient relationship by the state, by independent professional associations, by corporations, and by the direct force of the market. To take one illustration, when Parsons published *The Social System* more

than half a century ago (1951), his theory of the profession underpinned his notion of the sick role. He could assume the existence of an autonomous and self-regulating profession with a
virtually monopolistic control over the provision of medical
service and considerable influence over the university medical
curriculum. It was further assumed that patients felt trust and
were compliant with their doctors. Medical power meant that
the patient was required to embrace a medical regime in order
to reenter normal social relationships after a period of sickness.

The contrast between Parsons's idea of the professions in the
1950s and the present reality of doctoring in America and
Britain could hardly be greater (Derber 1984; Fryer 1991). For
example, British doctors went on unofficial strike on May 1,
2001, to protest working conditions. The overt purpose of the
strike was to draw attention to the overload of patients on
doctors' client lists, but deeper problems appear to be undermining the professional authority of the doctors and the
independent role of the British Medical Association. Another
recent case in Britain illustrates endemic problems of trust between doctors and patients: a fifty-eight-year-old woman alleged that during minor gynecological surgery in 1992, a
surgeon removed her healthy womb and ovaries without her
consent. *The Independent* reported in February 2000 that the
surgeon argued in court that during the operation he had found
a large irregular mass that could have been malignant, prompt-
ing the removal of the ovaries. In 2003, it was reported by Dr.
Jeremy Metters, the inspector of anatomy, that more than
twenty thousand brains had been removed from deceased patients for research purposes without the consent of relatives.
The problem is that in British law the Human Tissue Act does

not permit research on organs taken without consent, but it does not prevent it either. Patient trust and confidence in health delivery in general have been shaken by NHS shortages, by the postal-address lottery, by lack of consent in the removal of organs, by the case of Dr. Shipman, and by dead patients' being stored unceremoniously on the floor of overcrowded hospitals.

In Britain, the political attack on professional self-regulation was initiated by the Thatcher government, which attempted to promote the competitive market regulation of services by creating internal markets or quasi markets in the NHS. Both secondary and tertiary education systems have been transformed by a competitive and entrepreneurial culture that is incompatible with either a bureaucratic or a professional system. While these services have been simultaneously deregulated and deprofessionalized, they have also been subjected to regular auditing procedures. Successive British governments have imposed audit devices for setting standards, measuring performance, and rewarding success. The new regulatory devices that have been imposed on higher-education systems to measure research productivity and teaching outcomes, together with other student and peer reviews, are incompatible with professional self-regulation and autonomy. The profession is no longer an effective or significant regulatory body, and governments depend on a mixture of legal devices and market mechanisms. The disappearance of the professions as a topic of major sociological interest can itself be taken as a measure of the changing status of professions in social life.

The professions are not and cannot be effective regulatory devices in a global-risk society. As the scientific basis of economic production becomes more complex, both the public and the government depend on expert opinion. Paradoxically, this expert opinion itself is often divided, uncertain, and contradictory. Political scientists have concentrated primarily on the manipulation of medical and scientific opinion by multinational corporations; it is difficult to secure an independent and neutral analysis from scientific institutions owned largely by corporate interests (Waitzkin and Waterman 1974; Navarro 1986). For example, any attempt to test the long-term environmental effects of GM food production systematically will probably fail for political rather than scientific reasons. GM trials in Britain, according to *The Guardian* in October 2003, have shown that two GM crops grown experimentally—rapeseed and sugar beet—are harmful to the environment. In the context of international conflict, scientific arguments between private health and public health were often obscured by ideological conflicts. In the United States, defenders of socialized medicine during the cold war, such as the medical historian Henry E. Sigerist, were often regarded as dangerous Communists. While the collapse of Communism has made such debates look increasingly obsolete and peculiar, the role of corporate power in pharmaceutical research is clearly potent, as the failure of the Doha agreement and the international conflict over the price of HIV/AIDS treatment have demonstrated.

Another problem with scientific knowledge in the modern world is time. The pharmaceutical trials by which drugs are accepted as effective and safe are conducted within limited temporal boundaries that are ultimately determined by economic criteria. The long-term consequences of drugs on populations over generations are not included in commercial judgments

about efficacy, profitability, and safety. Moreover, it is difficult
to know about the effect of a drug or a chemical without trying
it out in a real setting over a long period. For example, we
know only in retrospect that dependence on insecticides in
postwar strategies to eradicate malaria in Africa and South Asia
has increased resistance to contemporary eradication programs.
As a result, malaria is increasing globally. The long-term effects of Prozac are also difficult to predict. What is the effect of
GM products on the social and natural environment over a
fifty-year period? While the FDA model for drug testing is
perfectly appropriate for medical products in the short term, it
does not attempt to measure their impact on human populations over generations. Because the time frame of a democrati-
cally elected government does not extend much beyond the
next election, it is difficult to secure the conditions for planning and policy formation over many decades.

Regulatory devices to manage the unintended risks of
medical innovation are imperfect because the traditional institutions of regulation (professions, universities, and government) are ineffective in the context of global competition.
Furthermore, contemporary scientific advice is increasingly
divided and incomplete because scientific knowledge is increasingly complex. The neutrality and the accuracy of expert
information are in question since the economic interests of corporations drive, manage, and orchestrate scientific debate.
Given the fragility of these institutional and scientific devices,
the global market has become the final arbiter of morals and
truth. Recent controversial cases—such as reproduction by a
wife who collected seed involuntarily from her unconscious
husband, who subsequently died from meningitis—have

shown that dissatisfied patients and clients will simply secure services on a global market. Government and intergovernmental arrangements to regulate organ transplants have failed because demand from patients has been robust and because there is a market to provide organs (such as kidneys) from criminals in China, who are executed once their organs have been surgically removed. It would require powerful international agreements to regulate this trade, but it is fairly certain that an illegal market in organs could never be wholly controlled. Government attempts to prevent human cloning will be circumvented by doctors, patients, or corporations that can find viable global solutions outside the legislative and moral norms of a local society or state. Recent attempts to distinguish between cloning of humans and therapeutic cloning of cells will be equally difficult to define and enforce by professions or governments. The scientific charisma (or at least notoriety) that will accrue to the scientist who clones the first human being will prove difficult to resist in a scientific environment driven by global competition, media interest, and the scientific celebrity system. The person who is so cloned will become, like Dolly, an icon of medical innovation and scientific progress.

TECHNOLOGY, LAW, AND THE BODY

The sociological study of risk could easily drive one to pessimistic conclusions, but we should not assume that all unanticipated consequences are bad (M. Douglas and Wildavsky 1982). Human rights legislation, global communication, and the Olympic Games are just as much consequences of globalization as online pornography and the decline of the common toad. One response to the risks of unregulated cloning, organ transplants, and reproductive technologies would be the creation of international law that can exercise some constraint over the intended and unintended effects of medical and scientific globalization. Martha Nussbaum's capability model attempts to spell out some basic guidelines for development programs to fulfill human capabilities, especially those of women (2000). Nussbaum drew on a raft of international legislation that attempts to enforce basic human rights. While such legislative agreements are constantly undermined and corrupted, they do provide a common starting point for the creation of a safer world.

In the absence of effective professional and market regulation, we need some political governance of medical technology. The consequences of a deregulated global market in organ transplants, drugs, and technologies would be catastrophic, but placing our hope in international legal constraints may be utopian. It has proved difficult or impossible to regulate the illicit trade in drugs. A political economist could persuasively claim that the economic power of global corporations working within or outside the law will determine the future of medical technology and that the rate of innovation in cloning will be a function of its profitability. To these arguments, there is at least one modest reply worth developing. Max Weber, in his sociology of the law, recognized that a capitalist economic system could not function without a legal framework (Turner 1981). A dynamic and unstable economic environment requires the stability of a legal administrative machine in order to secure the unimpeded exchange of commodities. In particular, global corporations require laws to enforce contracts, secure intellectual property, protect themselves against fraud and force, regulate competition, and provide some legal security for their assets. While corporations are obviously driven by an economic logic of profitability, they have a very real interest in legal enforcement. They will object to regulation politically, but they have no real advantage in unregulated risk. At the very least, they will need laws and courts within which to settle their own disputes. This legal condition of exchange provides the basis for global governance, and hence the proponents of classical models of liberal society—such as F. A. Hayek in *The Road to Serfdom* (1944), who regarded collective planning as incompatible with individual liberties—recognized that "the rule of law" was a necessary condition of individual and market freedom. Maintaining social order requires some legal and cultural constraints; otherwise, the use of fraud and force are rational strategies in a free market of competitive individuals (Parsons 1937).

MEDICAL CITIZENSHIP

Although human rights legislation in the twentieth century played an important part in world health measures, sociologists have neglected human rights institutions as a topic of research. One reason for that is that rights raise moral questions, which sociology, as a positive science, cannot easily answer (Sjoberg, Gill, and Williams 2001). By contrast, sociology has developed an articulate and compelling notion of citizenship in terms of a concept of social rather than human rights (Turner 1993, 1997a, 2001a). Given the dangers and opportunities of medical technology, social and human rights to health have become a major aspect of modern political struggle. In Western societies,

health is now regarded, often reluctantly and with qualification, as a social entitlement, but it can be satisfied only where
social resources have been redistributed without damage to
economic growth. The fundamental problems of the medical
economy are, like those of any economy, problems about scarce
resources, and scarcity creates divisions and competition, but
the existence of any human society requires social solidarity or
social capital. Social capital is a spontaneous and unplanned
consequence of social interconnectedness, but it requires the
support and protection of a legal framework, including one en-
suring social and human rights.

There is a contradiction between social solidarity and
scarcity. In the social sciences, these contradictory principles
are described as the allocative and integrative requirements of
social systems (Parsons 1951). Scarcity is particularly important in the medical economy because in developed societies,
affluence, lifestyle, and consumerism have magnified expectations of health and longevity. The baby boomers who are currently in their late middle age, grew up in a period in which
consumer culture did not expect them to grow old or retire.
This boomer generation will make considerable demands on
health care in the next two or three decades because they have
very high expectations of personal appearance and health and
the ability of scientific medicine to provide solutions to aging
(Edmunds and Turner 2002). The mirage of health has had the
paradoxical consequence of making health scarce in advanced
societies because expectation has outstripped the supply of effective cures and treatments. Health is seen as a social right in
modern societies, and therefore any sociological analysis of
health and illness in modernity must consider the impact of

social rights on the distribution of scarce resources.

Social citizenship provides a form of secular solidarity in response to economic scarcities and is an essential precondition for the development of social capital, but social cohesion is threatened by the inevitable presence of social inequality. In Durkheim's terms, social solidarity is eroded by the anomic conditions that include egoistic individualism, inequality, and isolation. The elastic demand for health illustrates the social and political tension between scarcity and solidarity. Health is a desirable, infinite, scarce resource in the context of the political changes to welfare institutions following the adoption of neoconservative economic strategies in the global economy. Health demands are infinitely elastic because the modern notion of health now covers all aspects of life and is inflated by consumer needs that are in turn swelled by advertising. Health is an expectation that is deeply embedded in our notion of lifestyle in consumer culture. Because social expectations are inflated by norms of activism, success, personal beauty, and youthfulness, disappointment is a necessary consequence of a consumer society, and disappointment is a definite, if submerged, feature of anomie. The paradox is that disappointment expands with affluence and creates the social conditions that foster unhappiness. This paradoxical link between affluence and disappointment partly explains the connections between economic growth, the decline in social capital, unhappiness, and poor health. The expansion of citizenship is one solution to the decline of social interconnectedness because citizenship expands the opportunities for social participation, involvement, and membership. In one sense, social policies actually make citizens by creating the conditions for their empowerment and self-realization. The political activism of lobbies representing the elderly in America is one illustration (Campbell 2003).

Social citizenship functions as an indispensable basis for social solidarity by alleviating the genetic legacy that predisposes individuals to disease and by mitigating the social causes of sickness, such as class and status inequalities. From the sociological perspective on social capital, health is the often unintended or disguised consequence of the social rights of citizenship rather than an intended outcome of technical and medical interventions. The germ theory of disease is a persuasive account of why we suffer from disease and sickness, but its very success as a causal story obscures the role of social and political conditions in good health. The argument in support of social capital as a general theory of health is supported by the growth of chronic conditions in modern societies because the management of chronicity requires the political input of long-term social resources.

Preventive health and social security measures improve the social environment of individuals, and their health characteristics will consequently improve. As social citizenship and entitlements expand, however, demands for health services are inevitably extended. Expectations will tend to be inflationary in an electoral democracy, where political parties compete for public support. As expectations rise and inflationary demands exceed welfare provisions, including medical capacities, scarcity is reintroduced. If disappointment is an inevitable consequence of rising expectations, individuals are unlikely to be satisfied with existing services, especially when those services are constrained by economic restrictions. Consumers of public health services will turn to alternative forms of supply, such as self-help groups, self-medication, and alternative medicine. Given the decline of professional monopolies over medical services, these political and economic conditions will tend to produce medical pluralism. The differentiation of medical and welfare services can cater to differences in medical needs, but differentiated medical care cannot guarantee fairness in the provision of services.

Citizenship institutions protect individuals from the negative consequences of the economic market in a capitalist society, particularly from the consequences of industrial injury, unemployment, sickness, and early retirement, but only if employee rights are supported by the law. The redistributive functions of citizenship institutions are the basis for justice because public goods are funded by a system of universal taxation that influences the whole population. Justice in this sense is fairness, and social arrangements are fair if there are no unjustifiable grounds for discrimination among members of a society (Rawls 1970). In this model, social arrangements are fair if the basic liberties of the individual are not constrained by the freedom of other members of society. Socioeconomic inequality exists only if it can be reasonably expected to benefit the position of the least advantaged. This liberal view of society—characteristic of such philosophers as Isaiah Berlin, F. A. Hayek, and John Rawls—defends negative rather than positive liberties; it is concerned with freedom from oppression and mistreatment rather than with the institution of positive liberties to achieve certain desirable outcomes. Citizenship attempts to reconcile individual rights (rights to free speech, for example) with collective rights (such as freedom from racial discrimination) within a democratic framework. In terms of health rights in a

democracy, individual liberties (such as personal sexual preferences) have to be reconciled with collective health safeguards
(from the unanticipated spread of HIV/AIDS and hepatitis, for
instance). Individual rights to health care must be negotiated
within these collective parameters of redistributive justice.

Because citizenship controls access to the scarce resources of
a society, the allocative function is often the basis for a profound conflict in modern societies, over criteria of citizenship
membership. In a democracy, social membership is a precondition for sharing in social resources, and therefore the legal conditions for the naturalization of aliens tell us a great deal about
the character of democracy in a society. These political and legal processes relate fundamentally to the basic notions of social
inclusion and exclusion. The willingness of communities to
share access to welfare and health care is a sensitive measure of
the extent of universal social rights. In legislative terms,
nation-states are generally reluctant to embrace new citizens
without some checks on their age, health status, and criminal
record. These processes of inclusion and exclusion mark both
the political and the moral boundaries of society. Moral panic
about the international spread of HIV/AIDS through tourism,
international trade, and other means is an important indicator
of cultural risk in a global context (O'Neill 1990). The SARS
epidemic has raised important issues about political secrecy
and the absence of effective democratic structures in China.
The failure of the Chinese authorities to respond openly and
quickly to evidence of a new virus fueled the subsequent panic
in Hong Kong and the rapid export of the virus to Vietnam,
Singapore, and Canada. Financial instability in Asia in 2003
was a consequence of the political failure to respond quickly

and transparently to SARS.

Social closure is an elementary form of group solidarity, producing both social bonding and inevitable alienation and stigmatization of outsiders. The legal boundaries of the state produce an enduring crisis for marginal communities in an ethnically plural society. In this negative sense, citizenship is about the surveillance and policing of normative borders (Connolly 1995). Any benchmark of citizenship would have to include some notion of egalitarian openness to difference and otherness as an essential ingredient of liberal democracy. Who gets citizenship indicates the prevailing criteria of inclusion and exclusion within a political community, and the way these social and economic resources are allocated and administered largely determines the economic fate of individuals and their families. From a historical perspective, the normative boundaries of society are defined by tolerance of outsiders—a tolerance that is typically limited and in which cultural difference is often defined in terms of medical issues, such as bubonic plague and leprosy in medieval times, by tuberculosis in the Victorian age, or by the contemporary spread of superbugs. In a global environment, the sacred and profane dichotomy that informed Durkheim's understanding of social connectedness is increasingly defined as a dichotomy between health and illness, where quarantine defines the moral and the medical simultaneously. With the advent of global biological terrorism, the anthrax attack in the United States is a clear illustration of how disease and the threat of disease can challenge national political boundaries and a society's vision of civilized behavior, because these biological threats require a global solution.

In the context of economic deregulation and neoconservatism in the 1980s and 1990s, there was an assumption that individuals must be made responsible for their own health and that they should not depend, as Thatcher argued, on the "nanny state." Preventive health campaigns promote the idea that we should practice "safe sex," especially with strangers, and that we should avoid risky behavior associated with smoking, alcohol, or lifestyle drugs. This emphasis on individual responsibility and self-care has emerged as a response to scarcity. Because chronic disease is such a crucial part of health-care and welfare budgets, doctors need to pay more attention to lifestyle in understanding and treating disease (Hansen 2001). With the increasing longevity of the populations of Western societies, the burden of dependency (the ratio of children and elderly to the working population) has a major impact on national budgets. There is growing awareness that very few Western governments have made adequate provision for the care of the elderly and many pension arrangements cannot be effectively funded through existing means. Public policy has responded by stressing individual responsibility, connecting work to welfare, and encouraging relatives to fund the retirement of their senior family members. These changes in public health philosophy encouraged the values of voluntarism and inevitably promote the idea that the family should be more involved in the care of its members. This preventive ethic places an increasing burden on health care from often-unemployed women and single mothers. The reduction of state support for health care has transferred the burden of care to women, the family, kinship networks, voluntary associations, and the local community. Against such a trend, some sociologists have argued that we have a right not to depend on the traditional charity of the family and kinship (Finch 1989). One consequence of policy changes with respect to welfare and health care is an inevitable increase in social inequality between educated professional groups and the unskilled, manual working class. Voluntary or community provision of health care should not attempt to be, and can never be, universalistic because associational forms of health delivery are normally directed at a specific, not a general, clientele.

The question of family obligation raises the issue of changing forms of social involvement and entitlement. The early stages in the development of citizenship appeared to depend on the unrecognized contributions of women, who were outside the paid labor market but involved in domestic labor. The conventional patterns of citizenship have depended on a Fordist economy, which assumes that men work to generate income to sustain their own domestic arrangements and to provide, through retirement savings, for the future of their household. Within such an economic system, women are assumed to provide domestic labor for men and to reproduce society through motherhood and care of their children. Social contract theory reproduced the dominant assumptions of patriarchy, which depend on this public-private division. Women's unpaid domestic labor was thus fundamental to the maintenance of the external political structures of national citizenship. The historical relegation of women to the private domain of the nuclear family created permanent dependency and made their formal entry into the labor market after their children had left home problematic. This pattern of citizenship contributed to the social isolation and invisibility of women.

These assumptions of a Fordist economy have been transformed by global changes in the labor market—with casualization, computerization in production and distribution, the increase in female employment, changes to the family, the feminization of poverty in single-parent families—and by changes to retirement legislation. The conventional and simple division between the private and public realms has been transformed by social changes. The consequences for health and health care are considerable.

EQUALITY AND HEALTH

In employing health as an index of social rights, we need to distinguish between morbidity rates (the statistics on illness and disease in both acute and chronic conditions) and mortality rates (the pattern and causes of death over time). The improvement in mortality rates (especially from infectious diseases among children) in the nineteenth and early twentieth centuries was largely a result of improvements in the standard of living (diet, water supply, education, and housing) rather than a direct consequence of medical intervention (McKeown 1979; Turner 1995a). These historical arguments can be used to demonstrate that an increase in life expectancy from birth is a general index of citizenship because an improvement in the social environment reduces infant mortality. These debates are part of the legacy of social and political reform, in which democracy and the redistribution of resources by taxation are seen to be the most effective social response to the existence of disease (Gerhardt 1989; Siegrist 2000). This argument, which is controversial, is the basic plank of the political-economy perspective on health and illness.

As we have seen in this study, there is a significant amount of sociological research on the relationship between social class and health (Navarro and Berman 1977). In the United Kingdom, the Black Report in 1980 (Townsend and Davidson 1982), "The Health Divide" (Whitehead 1988), and Will Hutton's *New Life for Health* (2000) demonstrated an almost perfect match between the socioeconomic position and life expectancy (Blane 1985; Macintyre 1997). The research of Richard Wilkinson (1986, 1996) has shown the persistence of the connection between social class inequalities and illness and the comparative importance of the welfare state in explaining better health outcomes in Scandinavian societies. The comparative research of Ichiro Kawachi and Bruce Kennedy in *The Health of Nations* (2002) has shown that the American experience of inequality and health is no exception. There is a scientific consensus that social class is crucial in the production of inequalities in morbidity and mortality, but there has been considerable debate about how the relationship between socioeconomic deprivation and illness should be understood. The class and health relationships are complicated by gender, ethnicity, and age (Krieger et al. 1993). Women generally live longer than men but experience higher levels of morbidity (Arber 1997; Arber and Cooper 2000; Arber and Thomas 2001). There are important gender divisions in terms of both physical and mental health; these differences are primarily connected to different patterns of employment, social involvement, social status, and lifestyle (Busfield 2000). Some differences between men and women may be related to variations in sickness reporting, but improvements in female health have been associated with a decline in female fertility, improvements in the management of reproduction, and changes in education. In short, health in women is associated with the improvement in their social rights as a result of political lobbying by the women's movement and other social forces. As we have seen in earlier chapters, there is also evidence that as women enter the labor force in significant numbers and leave traditional nurturing roles, they acquire the health profile of men.

A similar set of arguments applies to aging. There was a significant increase in life expectancy for both men and women in Western societies throughout the last century. These improvements point to a general expansion of social welfare through citizenship institutions in terms of retirement benefits, income support, and health care. While we live longer, however, morbidity data show a corresponding increase in patterns of chronic illness. There is a significant increase in the prevalence of disability for men and women over the age of sixty-five, and in United States, 22 percent of this age group require some form of assistance to accomplish daily tasks (Albrecht 1992).

There has also been a significant change in the epidemiological profile of society and a distinct increase in deaths from degenerative disease (in particular, from cancers, strokes, and heart failure). Infectious diseases have increased with globalization; WHO has shown that whereas noncommunicable diseases represented 43 percent of all disease in 1998, the proportion rose to 73 percent by 2002. Because these diseases primarily have social causes, there is pressure to seek social solutions to this epidemiological transition. In the United Kingdom, breast cancer is now the most important cause of death among women past menopause. These developments are a result of the aging of the population and the decline in lung cancer following a reduction in smoking among men. Whether an improvement in citizenship alone can extend life expectancy and reduce chronic morbidity is a crucial question for public health in the next century. Epidemiological research suggests that once a certain level of affluence has been achieved, the genetic legacy of individuals plays an increasing role in the experiences of illness and disease. Yet there are puzzling and persistent cultural variations in terms of disease prevalence. For example, prostate and breast cancers are much lower in Japan than in the United States and Britain. These variations may be accounted for by differences in living conditions, dietary practices, and genetic legacy.

Nussbaum (2000, 78–80), in terms of "central human functional capabilities," has expressed the relationship between health, well-being, and social resources. The basic idea behind this model is that we should be able to develop universal criteria to make judgments about justice in terms of basic human functions. She provided a list of ten such capabilities: to live a life of normal length; to enjoy good health, including reproductive health; to enjoy bodily integrity (such as freedom from sexual assault); to use the senses (for imagination and reasoning); to form emotional relationships with other humans; to engage in critical reflection on one's life; to form effective and rewarding affiliations with other people; to sympathize with other species and exercise stewardship over their lives; to engage in play and to enjoy leisure; and to exercise some control over one's political and material environment. Nussbaum believes that these capabilities are universal and that they form the basic human rights, a range of rights that universally protect and enhance these capabilities. Recognition of these fundamental capabilities provides a moral framework for democratic governance and the dignity of human beings.

Nussbaum's capability approach throws further light on the importance of citizenship as a collection of social rights and, hence, as the framework within which people can expect a basic level of good health. Governments that fail to respect basic capabilities undermine the health and well-being of their citizens. Nussbaum's theory of capabilities has also been used to establish a basic legal framework for the protection of women and to ensure that women's capabilities are given equal respect by society. Where extreme forms of social inequality exist in a class or caste society, the capabilities of individuals cannot be equally achieved. Nussbaum has developed this approach to provide a general set of values that can direct policy and strategy for development, but her criteria of capability is equally valuable in assessing the success or failure of social policies designed to enhance health through social citizenship (Turner 1999b).

NEOCONSERVATISM AND ECONOMIC DEREGULATION

The historical relationships between health and citizenship were established by the expansion of welfare in the postwar period and by a general expansion of the economies of postwar industrial societies. Since the early 1980s, economic deregulation, privatization, and commodification, as well as changes in public policy toward unemployment, retirement, and health, have challenged these welfare arrangements. Governments in the United Kingdom and the United States no longer assume that full employment is a principal goal of economic policy. Contemporary governments are more likely to accept the economic argument that the growth in employment depends on the level of investment in markets that are not constrained by government regulation. It is also increasingly assumed that individuals will pay for welfare services (the "user-pays" doctrine), that society should protect itself from "free riders," and that the voluntary sector (such as the large charities and churches) will contribute significantly to the national welfare effort. It is also taken for granted that there will be a significant level of privatization in welfare, health care, and education. Welfare provision will be subject to the same controls and philosophy as industry itself. In the jargon of contemporary economic theory, the provision of services, whether by government or the voluntary sector, must conform to quality-control processes, auditing, case management, "one-stop shopping," outsourcing, and competitive funding models. It is unclear how great the impact of these changes on social rights will be in the long term, but it is clear that state provision of welfare will be increasingly relocated in the private sector.

We have seen that the majority of industrial societies in the postwar period experienced social reconstruction. After the ravages of warfare, many governments implicitly or explicitly adopted social-Keynesian policies for stimulating the economy through investments in health, education, housing, and other so-called infrastructural expenditures. In short, recovery was driven by investment in human capital. Following the social policies of Keynesian economics, governments attempted to control the level of unemployment through investments in public works, such as road building. Keynesianism was part of a more general philosophy arguing that the state, rather than the market, should be pivotal in providing for the needs of its citizens. In the United Kingdom, for example, the reports of William Beveridge, such as *Full Employment in a Free Society* (1944), provided a framework for the development of a health system that would regard the health needs of the nation as a citizen's right. In the United States, there were similar developments in the twentieth century, in the New Deal and Progressive Era (Milio 1985). In Canada, there was a parallel development of citizenship rights, social reconstruction, and universalistic healthcare reform (Redden 2002). In the 1970s and 1980s, the Keynesian philosophy of public support for health and welfare became unpopular as governments sought to reduce public expenditure, reduce personal taxation, and rely on market competition to drive down inflation. These policies have been adopted in the United States, the United Kingdom, Canada, New Zealand, and Australia.

Neoconservative policies attempt to increase the profitability of economic corporations by reducing their tax burden, removing legal constraints on their activities, and removing trade barriers. At the same time, laissez faire policies require individuals to take more responsibility for their own health care by adopting healthy lifestyles and providing for retirement through personal investments. Because these policies attempted to reduce state expenditure, there have been a variety of experiments to transfer responsibility for the provision of health and welfare services to community groups and voluntary associations. Although these partnerships between the voluntary and the state sectors can reduce welfare bureaucracy and bring services more directly to the client, the voluntary sector cannot produce a uniform or universal service, and many critics have argued that it is driven by the same logic as the market, namely, the principle of resource maximization (Brown, Kenny, and Turner 2000). The voluntary sector is less subject to quality control and efficiency measurements and is hence less accountable. Neoconservatism arose because of fears that corporate profitability had been eroded by taxation and government regulation of the economy and by the graying of the population. Partnerships between the voluntary sector and the state are often promoted not because they will create "active citizenship" but because some measure of voluntarism will reduce the public cost of welfare services. The consequences of neoconservatism are thought to be incompatible with the values of social equality that underpinned the creation of the postwar welfare state. While the health benefits of welfare-state expenditure were often disappointing insofar as they failed to remove the effects of class inequality, neoconservatism will have profoundly negative consequences for health.

Conclusion: Globalization, Citizenship, and Social Capital

The negative features of global neoconservatism were spelled out in an influential article by David Coburn (2000) on "Income Inequality, Social Cohesion, and Health Status of Populations." Coburn has argued that neoconservatism diminishes the authority of the state and makes it difficult for governments to achieve their welfare priorities. At the same time, it increases social inequality and reduces the level of social cohesion (or social capital) in society. These structural changes lower the level of social trust and diminish self-respect among members of those sectors exposed to growing social inequality. Low self-respect and declining social trust have a direct effect on health, by lowering immunity to illness. Coburn's approach is important because it allows us to make direct connections between the global growth of neoconservatism, the decline in social cohesion, and the erosion of the health of individuals.

These neoconservative changes suggest an important insight into the history of citizenship: social rights are not evolutionary or cumulative. Because T. H. Marshall (1963) argued that the rights of citizenship were cumulative, he also assumed that once the basic legal, political, and welfare rights had been achieved, they would not be easily eroded. He claimed that each of these historical stages represents a successful accumulation of citizenship. His is an overly optimistic picture of the historical evolution of rights. One of the important debates emerging in contemporary democracies is whether previously held rights, including the right to health, can be sustained in a society that is increasingly dominated by the needs of the marketplace and the rhetoric of economic rationalism. In a market-driven society, young people find it difficult to enter the labor market and gain access to resources because of the nature of the economy. If we regard full employment as an entitlement, social rights may be weakened as a consequence of economic rationalism. One can identify many societies that have highly developed social and economic rights but do not have adequate legal and political rights. The former Communist regimes of Eastern Europe institutionalized social and economic forms of citizenship, but legal and political rights were often absent. They had economic rights without a comprehensive civil society because they had achieved industrialization without a revolution against feudal privilege.

It is not clear how societies will manage the social conflicts that result from a failure to respect rights. Citizenship provides a form of solidarity—the social glue that binds together societies that are otherwise divided by social class, gender, ethnicity, and age. It functions as a basic form of social capital. This model of the history of citizenship has either optimistic or pessimistic implications. The optimistic view is that through the United Nations and through agreements on human rights, modern societies can manage the problem of interstate violence, terrorism, and conflict. The alternative view is that we do not, in fact, have cumulative citizenship; what we have is an erosion or breakdown of citizenship (Turner 1993). Many nation-states can no longer adequately provide the social rights of citizenship for their members because their scope for public policy implementation is constrained by the economic power of global corporations. As social capital is a necessary condition for both individual and collective health, the erosion of citizenship also erodes the social conditions that promote good health. Health, as a fundamental right, is a critical feature of political struggle.

In *The Sociological Imagination* (1959), the American sociologist C. Wright Mills (1959), famously said that the promise of sociology was to illuminate and explain the relationship between our personal troubles and public issues. More elegantly, he said that the sociological imagination sought to express and analyze the connections between biography and social structure. Troubles concern the individual while issues transcend local circumstances, and hence the sociologist must connect the local with the global. Knowledge of the relationship between biography and social structure can give us the capacity to change the relationship in order to make our troubles less burdensome. The promise of sociology is to enhance our freedom to act more wisely and prudently. In this study, I have followed Mills's excellent advice in trying to connect our personal experiences of illness as trouble to the larger canvas of the political economy of modern societies and the process of globalization.

Although we may visit a doctor infrequently, we are constantly bothered by medical troubles. These may be relatively minor irritations, such as constipation, earache, strained eyesight, or migraine. Whether these complaints are minor problems or major crises, we fall ill because we are embodied and vulnerable. We develop narratives of these troubles and find solace in them, but we need the social support that comes from viable social relationships if we are to survive the tribulations of disease and discomfort. The support of these social relations is the positive impact of social capital. Our troubles are made tolerable by the social networks that support us and the trust that arises from our social bonds, but these networks are constantly eroded by social change, and hence citizenship becomes a critical buttress of health and prosperity. Although Mills wrote an influential study of the power elite in America (1956), he did not study the medical establishment, medical power, and health inequalities. However, the problematic relationships between personal troubles, health and illness, the power of the medical elite in society, and the impact of the global economy perfectly illustrate his major concern: that the sociologist has a moral role to illuminate and criticize the social problems of the period in which he or she lives. Health inequality, poverty, and depression are pressing issues of modern society, and as sociologists we need to listen attentively to the narratives of private troubles if we are to grapple with the larger structures of political and economic power. The private narratives of illness tell a powerful story about the public issues of wealth, power, and status. They also tell us about the fortitude of people who constantly face their own human vulnerability and survive the experiences of illness and disease.

REFERENCES

Abercrombie, N., S. Hill, and B. S Turner. 1980. *The dominant ideology thesis.* London: George Allen & Unwin.

Albrecht, G. L. 1992. *The disability business: Rehabilitation in America.* Newbury Park, Calif.: SAGE.

Albrecht, G. L., R. Fitzpatrick, and S. C. Scrimshaw, eds. 2000. *The handbook of social studies in health and medicine.* London: SAGE.

Albrecht, G. L., K. D. Seelman, and M. Bury, eds. 2001. *Handbook of disability studies.* Thousand Oaks, Calif.: SAGE.

Albrecht, G. L., and L. M. Verbrugge. 2000. "The global experience of disability." In Albrecht, Fitzpatrick, and Scrimshaw 2000, 293–307.

Aleinikoff, T. A., and B. D. Klusmeyer, eds. 2000. *From migrants to citizens: Membership in a changing world.* Washington, D.C.: Carnegie Endowment for International Peace.

Alexander, J. 1994. "The return of civil society." *Contemporary Sociology* 27:797–803.

Altman, D. 2001. *Global sex.* Chicago: Univ. of Chicago Press.

Annandale, E., and K. Hunt, eds. 2000. *Gender inequalities in health.* Buckingham, U.K.: Open Univ. Press.

Antonucci, T. C., K. J. Ajrouch, and M. R. Janevic. 2003. "The effect of social relations with children on the education-health link in men and women aged forty and over." *Social Science & Medicine* 56 (5): 949–60.

Arber, S. 1997. "Comparing inequalities in women's and men's health: Britain in the 1990s." *Social Science & Medicine* 44 (6): 773–87.

Arber, S., and H. Cooper. 2000. "Gender and inequalities in health across the lifecourse." In *Gender inequalities in health*, ed. E. Annandale and K. Hunt, 123–49. Buckingham, U.K.: Open Univ. Press.

Arber, S., and H. Thomas. 2001. "From women's health to a gender analysis of health." In Cockerham 2001, 94–113.

Ariès, P., and A. Béjin, eds. 1985. *Western sexuality: Practice and precept in past and present times.* Trans. A. Forster. Oxford: Basil Blackwell.

315

Armstrong, D. 1983. *Political anatomy of the body: Medical knowledge in Britain in the twentieth century*. Cambridge: Cambridge Univ. Press.

Arnold, D. 2000. *The new Cambridge history of India: Science, technology, and medicine in colonial India*. Cambridge: Cambridge Univ. Press.

Atchley, R. C. 1989. "A continuity theory of normal aging." *Gerontologist* 29 (2): 183–90.

Auslander, G. K., and N. Gold. 1999. "Disability terminology in the media: A comparison of newspaper reports in Canada and Israel." *Social Science & Medicine* 48 (10): 1395–1405.

Axford, B. 1995. *The global system: Economics, politics, and culture*. Cambridge: Polity Press.

Axtman, R. 1996. *Liberal democracy into the twenty-first century: Globalization integration and the nation-state*. Manchester, U.K.: Manchester Univ. Press.

Baks, K. 1991. "The 'eclipse' of folk medicine in Western society." *Sociology of Health & Illness* 13 (1): 20–38.

Ballard, K. D., D. J. Kuh, and M. E. J. Wadsworth. 2001. "The role of the menopause in women's experience of the 'change of life.' " *Sociology of Health & Illness* 23 (4): 397–424.

Balsam, A. 1995. "Forms of technological embodiment: Reading the body in contemporary culture." In *Cyberspace, cyberbodies, cyberpunk: Cultures of technological embodiment*, ed. M. Featherstone and R. Burrows, 215–37. London: SAGE.

Barbalet, J. 1998. *Emotion, social theory, and social structure: A macrosociological approach*. Cambridge: Cambridge Univ. Press.

Barker, K. K. 1998. "A ship upon a stormy sea: The medicalization of pregnancy." *Social Science & Medicine* 47 (8): 1067–76.

Barnes, C., G. Mercer, and T. Shakespeare. 1999. *Exploring disability: A sociological introduction*. Cambridge: Polity Press.

Bauböck, R. 1994. *Transnational citizenship: Membership rights in international migration*. Aldershot, U.K.: Edward Elgar.

Beck, U. 1992. *Risk society: Towards a new modernity*. Trans. M. Ritter. London: SAGE. (Orig. pub. 1986.)

Beck, U., and E. Beck-Gernsheim. (1995) *The Normal Chaos of Love*. Trans. M. Ritter and J. Wiebel. Cambridge: Polity Press. (Orig. pub. 1990.)

Becker, G. 1997. *Disrupted lives: How people create meaning in a chaotic world*. Berkeley: Univ. of California Press.

Becker, H. S., B. Geer, E. C. Hughes, and A. L. Strauss. 1961. *The boys in white: Student culture in medical school*. Chicago: Univ. of Chicago Press.

Bell, D., and J. Binnie. 2002. "Sexual citizenship: Marriage, the market and the military." In Richardson and Seidman 2002, 443–57.

Berger, P. L. 1963. *Invitation to Sociology*. Garden City, N.Y.: Doubleday.

———. 1969. *The social reality of religion*. London: Faber & Faber.

———. 1980. Foreword to *Man in an age of technology* by Arnold Gehlen. New York: Columbia Univ. Press.

———. 1998. *The limits of social cohesion: Conflict and mediation in pluralist societies*. Boulder, Colo.: Westview Press.

Berger, P. L., and H. Kellner. 1965. "Arnold Gehlen and the theory of institutions." *Social Research* 32 (1): 110–13.

Berger, P. L., and T. Luckmann. 1966. *The social construction of reality: A treatise in the sociology of knowledge*. Garden City, N.Y.: Doubleday.

Berkman, L. F. 1995. "The role of social relations in health promotion." *Psychosomatic Medicine* 57:245–54.

Berkman, L. F., and T. Glass. 2000. "Social integration, social networks, social support, and health." In Berkman and Kawachi 2000, 137–73.

Berkman, L. F., T. Glass, I. Brissette, and T. E. Seeman. 2000. "From social integration to health: Durkheim in the new millennium." *Social Science & Medicine* 51 (6): 843–57.

Berkman, L. F., and I. Kawachi, eds. 2000. *Social epidemiology*. New York: Oxford Univ. Press.

Berkman, L. F., L. Leo-Summers, and R. I. Horwitz. 1992. "Emotional support and survival following myocardial infarction: A prospective population-based study of the elderly." *Annals of Internal Medicine* 117:1003–9.

Berkman, S. L., and S. L. Syme. 1979. "Social networks, host resistance, and mortality: A nine-year follow-up study of Alameda County residents." *American Journal of Epidemiology* 109:186–204.

Berlin, I. 1979. *Four essays on liberty*. Oxford: Oxford Univ. Press.

Berliner, H. S. 1984. "Scientific medicine since Flexner." In *Alternative medicine: Popular and policy prespectives*, ed. J. W. Salmon, 30–56. London: Tavistock.

Beveridge, W. H. 1944. *Full employment in a free society*. London: George Allen & Unwin.

Beyer, P. 1994. *Religion and globalization*. London: SAGE.

Bickenbach, J. E. 1993. *Physical disability and social policy*. Toronto: Univ. of Toronto Press.

Bickenbach, J. E., S. Chatterji, E. M. Bailey, and T. B. Ustun. 1999. "Models of disablement, universalism, and the international classification of impairments, disabilities, and handicaps." *Social Science & Medicine* 48 (9): 1173–88.

Blane, D. 1985. "An assessment of the Black Report's explanation of health inequalities." *Sociology of Health and Illness* 7 (3): 423–45.

Blaxter, M. 2000. "Medical sociology at the start of the new millennium." *Social Science & Medicine* 51 (8): 1139–42.

Bordo, S. 1993. *Unbearable weight: Feminism, Western culture, and the body*. Berkeley: Univ. of California Press.

Bourdieu, P. 1990. *The logic of practice*. Cambridge: Polity Press.

———. 1993. *Sociology in question*. London: SAGE.

Brah, A., M. J. Hickman, M. Mac an Ghaill. 1999. *Global futures: Migration, environment, and globalization*. London: Macmillan.

Brown, G. W., and T. Harris. 1978. *Social origins of depression*. London: Tavistock.

Brown, K., S. Kenny, and B. S. Turner. 2000. *Rhetorics of welfare: Uncertainty, choice, and voluntary associations*. Basingstoke, U.K.: Macmillan.

Bruch, H. 1978. *The golden cage: The enigma of anorexia nervosa*. Cambridge, Mass.: Harvard Univ. Press.

Bruch, H. 1988. *Conversations with anorexics*. New York: Basic Books.

Brumberg, J. J. 1988. *Fasting girls: The emergence of anorexia nervosa as a modern disease*. Cambridge, Mass.: Harvard Univ. Press.

Buelens, F., ed. 1999. *Globalisation and the nation-state*. Cheltenham, U.K.: Edward Elgar.

Burchell, G., C. Gordon, and P. Miller, eds. 1991. *The Foucault effect: Studies in governmentality*. London: Harvester Wheatsheaf.

Bury, M. 1982. "Chronic illness as biographical disruption." *Sociology of Health & Illness* 4 (2): 167–82.

Busfield, J. 2000. "Rethinking the sociology of mental health." *Sociology of Health & Illness* 22 (5): 543–58.

Bynum, C. W. 1991. *Fragmentation and redemption: Essays on gender and the human body in medieval religion*. New York: Zone Books.

Cabezas, A. L. 2002. "Tourism, sex work, and women's rights in the Dominican Republic." In *Globalization and human rights*, ed. A. Brysk, 44–60. Berkeley: Univ. of California Press.

Campbell, A. L. 2003. *How policies make citizens: Senior political activism and the American welfare state*. Princeton, N.J.: Princeton Univ. Press.

Case, R. B., A. J. Moss, and N. Case. 1992. "Living alone after myocardial infarction." *Journal of the American Medical Association* 267:515–19.

Caskey, N. 1986. "Interpreting anorexia nervosa." In *The female body in Western culture: Contemporary perspectives,* ed. S. R. Suleiman, 175–89. Cambridge, Mass.: Harvard Univ. Press.

Charmaz, K. 1994. "Identity dilemmas of chronically ill men." *Sociological Quarterly* 35 (2): 269–88.

Chernin, K. 1981. *The obsession: Reflections on the tyranny of slenderness*. New York: Harper & Row.

Clarke, J. N. 1983. "Sexism, feminism, and medicalism: A decade review of literature on gender and illness." *Sociology of Health & Illness* 5 (1): 62–82.

Clendening, L., ed. 1942. *Source book of medical history*. Mineola, N.Y.: Dover.

Coburn, D. 2000. "Income inequality, social cohesion, and the health status of populations: The role of neo-liberalism." *Social Science & Medicine* 51 (1): 139–50.

Cockerham, W. C. 1986. *Medical sociology*. Englewood Cliffs, N.J.: Prentice Hall.

———. 2000. "Health lifestyles in Russia." *Social Science & Medicine* 51 (9): 1313–24.

———. 2001. *The Blackwell companion to medical sociology*. Oxford: Basil Blackwell.

Coleman, J. S. 1988. "Social capital in the creation of human capital." *American Journal of Sociology* 94:S95–S120.

———. 1994. *Foundations of social theory.* Cambridge, Mass.: Harvard Univ. Press, Belknap Press.

Connolly, W. E. 1995. *Two ethos of pluralization.* Minneapolis: University of Minnesota Press.

Conrad, P. 1992. "Medicalisation and social control." *Annual Review of Sociology* 18:209–32.

Conrad, P., and M. Bury. 1997. "Anselm Strauss and the sociological study of chronic illness: A reflection and appreciation." *Sociology of Health & Illness* 19 (3): 373–76.

Conrad, P., and J. Gabe. 1999. "Sociological perspectives on the new genetics: An overview." *Sociology of Health & Illness* 21 (5): 597–621.

Corbin, J. M., and A. L. Strauss. 1987. "Accompaniments of chronic illness: Changes in body, self, biography, and biographical time." In *The experience and management of chronic illness.* Vol. 6 of *Research in the sociology of health care,* ed. J. A. Roth and P. Conrad, 249–81. Greenwich, Conn.: JAI Press.

———. 1988. *Unending work and care: Managing chronic illness at home.* San Francisco: Jossey-Bass.

Corea, G. 1985. *The mother machine: Reproductive technologies from artificial insemination to artificial wombs.* New York: Harper & Row.

Coulter, H. L. 1977. *Divided legacy: A history of the schism in medical thought.* 2 vols. Washington, D.C.: Wehawken Books.

Cowan, J. K., M. B. Dembour, and R. A. Wilson, eds. 2001. *Culture and rights: Anthropological perspectives.* Cambridge: Cambridge Univ. Press.

Crossley, M. L. 2003. " 'Let me explain': Narrative emplotment and one patient's experience of oral cancer." *Social Science & Medicine* 56 (3): 439–48.

Crisp, A. H., R. L. Palmer, and R. S. Kalucy. 1976. "How common is anorexia nervosa? A prevalence study." *British Journal of Psychiatry* 128:549–54.

Cumming, E. 1963. "Further thoughts on the theory of disengagement." *International Social Science* 15:377–93.

Cumming, E., and W. E. Henry. 1961. *Growing old: The process of disengagement.* New York: Basic Books.

Cunningham, A. 1997. *The anatomical renaissance: The resurrection of the anatomical projects of the ancients.* Aldershot, U.K.: Scolar Press.

Dasgupta, P. 1993. *An inquiry into well-being and destitution.* Oxford: Clarendon Press.

Dasgupta, P., and I. Serageldin, eds. 2000. *Social capital: A multifaceted perspective.* Washington, D.C.: World Bank.

Davey Smith, G. 1996. "Income inequality and morality: Why are they related?" *British Medical Journal,* 312:987–88.

Davidson, J. 2000. "A phenomenology of fear: Merleau-Ponty and agoraphobic lifeworlds." *Sociology of Health & Illness* 22 (6): 640–60.

Davies, M. 1997. "Shattered assumptions: Time and the experience of long-term HIV positivity." *Social Science & Medicine* 44 (5): 561–71.

Davis, F. 1963. *Passage through crisis: Polio victims and their families*. Indianapolis, Ind.: Bobbs-Merrill.

Davis, K. 1995. *Reshaping the female body*. New York: Routledge.

———. 2002. " 'A dubious equality': Men, women, and cosmetic surgery." *Body & Society* 8 (1): 49–65.

Davis, L. J. 1996. *Enforcing normalcy: Disability, deafness, and the body*. London: Verso.

Deegan, M. J. 1978. "Living and acting in an altered body: A phenomenological description of amputation." *Journal of Sociology & Social Welfare* 5 (3): 342–55.

Derber, C. 1984. "Physicians and their sponsors: The new medical relations of production." In *Issues in the political economy of health*, ed. J. B. McKinlay, 217–54. London: Tavistock.

Dohrenwend, B. S., and B. P. Dohrenwend, eds. 1981. *Stressful life events and their context*. New York: Prodist.

Dormandy, T. 1999. *The white death: The history of tuberculosis*. London: Hambledon Press.

Douglas, J. D. 1967. *The social meanings of suicide*. Princeton, N.J.: Princeton Univ. Press.

Douglas, M. 1966. *Purity and danger: An analysis of concepts of pollution and tabu*. London: Routledge & Kegan Paul.

———. 1992. *Risk and blame: Essays in cultural theory*. London: Routledge.

Douglas, M., and A. Wildavsky. 1982. *Risk and culture: An essay on the selection of technical and environmental dangers*. Berkeley: Univ. of California Press.

Doyle, D., G. W. C. Hanks, and N. MacDonald, eds. 1998. *Oxford textbook of palliative care*. Oxford: Oxford Univ. Press.

Dubos, R. 1960. *Mirage of health: Utopias, progress, and biological change*. London: George Allen & Unwin.

Due, P., B. Holstein, R. Lund, J. Modvig, and K. Avlund. 1999. "Social relations, network, support, and relational strain." *Social Science & Medicine* 48 (5): 661–73.

Durkheim, E. 1951. *Suicide: A Study in sociology*. Trans. J. A. Spaulding and G. Simpson. Glencoe, Ill.: Free Press. (Orig. pub. 1897.)

———. 1954. *The Elementary forms of the religious life*. Trans. J. W. Swain. London: George Allen & Unwin. (Orig. pub. 1912.)

———. 1964. *The rules of sociological method*. Trans. S. S. Solovay and J. H. Mueller. New York: Free Press. (Orig. pub. 1895.)

———. 1992. *Professional ethics and civic morals*. Trans. C. Brookfield. London: Routledge.

Durkheim, E., and M. Mauss. 1963. *Primitive classification*. Trans. R. Needham. Chicago: Chicago Univ. Press. (Orig. pub. 1903.)

Eckersley, R., and K. Dear. 2002. "Cultural correlates of youth suicide." *Social Science & Medicine* 55 (11): 1891–1904.

Eder, K. 1996. *The social construction of nature*. London: SAGE.

Edmunds, J., and B. S. Turner. 2002. *Generations, culture, and society*. Buckingham, U.K.: Open Univ. Press.

Ehrenreich, B., and J. Ehrenreich. 1970. *The American health empire: Power, profits, and policies*. New York: Random House.

Ehrenreich, B., and D. English. 1973. *Complaints and disorders: the sexual politics of sickness*. Old Westbury, N.Y.: Feminist Press.

———. 1978. *For her own good: 150 years of the experts' advice to women*. New York: Anchor Books.

Eisner, M. A. 1993. *Regulatory politics in transition*. Baltimore: John Hopkins Univ. Press.

Elias, N. 1978. *The history of manners*. Vol. 1 of *The civilizing process*. Trans. E. Jephcott. Oxford: Basil Blackwell.

———. 1982. *The loneliness of the dying*. Trans. E. Jephcott. Oxford: Basil Blackwell.

Erickson, R. A. 1997. *The language of the heart: 1600–1750*. Philadelphia: Univ. of Pennsylvania Press.

Evans, D. 1993. *Sexual citizenship: The material construction of sexualities*. London: Routledge.

Ezzy, D. 2000. "Illness narratives: Time, hope, and HIV." *Social Science & Medicine* 50 (5): 605–17.

Featherstone, M., ed. 2000. *Body modification*. London: SAGE.

Featherstone, M., S. Lash, and R. Robertson, eds. 1995. *Global modernities*. London: SAGE.

Featherstone, M., and A. Wernick, eds. 1995. *Images of aging: Cultural representations of later life*. London: Routledge.

Fee, E., and T. M. Brown, eds. 1997. *Making medical history: The life and times of Henry E. Sigerist*. Baltimore: Johns Hopkins Univ. Press.

Finch, J. 1989. *Family obligations and social change*. Cambridge: Polity Press.

Findlay, M. 2000. *The globalisation of crime: Understanding transitional relationships in context*. Cambridge: Cambridge Univ. Press.

Fiscella, K., and P. Franks. 1997. "Poverty or income inequality as a predictor of mortality: Longitudinal cohort study." *British Medical Journal* 314:1724–28.

Fleming, C. 2002. "Performance as guerrilla ontology: The case of Stelarc." *Body & Society* 8 (3): 95–109.

Flexner, A. 1910. *Medical education in the United States and Canada*. New York: Carnegie Foundation for the Advancement of Teaching.

Foss, L., and K. Rothenberg. 1987. *The second medical revolution—From biomedicine to infomedicine*. London: Shambhala.

Foucault, M. 1970. *The order of things: An archaeology of the human sciences*. London: Tavistock. (Orig. pub. 1966.)

———. 1971. *Madness and civilisation: A history of insanity in the age of reason*. Trans. R. Howard. London: Tavistock. (Orig. pub. 1961.)

———. 1973. *The birth of the clinic: An archaeology of medical perception*. Trans. A. M. Sheridan-Smith. London: Tavistock. (Orig. pub. 1963.)

———. 1977. *Discipline and punish: The birth of the prison.* Trans. A. M. Sheridan-Smith. London: Tavistock. (Orig. pub. 1975.)

———. 1979. *An Introduction.* Vol. 1 of *The history of sexuality.* Trans. R. Hurley. London: Allen Lane. (Orig. pub. 1976.)

———. 1980a. *Power/knowledge: Selected interviews and other writings, 1972–1977.* Trans. C. Gordon. Brighton, U.K.: Harvester Wheatsheaf.

———. 1980b. *Herculine Barbin: Being the recently discovered memoirs of a nineteenth-century French hermaphrodite.* Trans. R. McDougall. Brighton, U.K.: Harvester. (Orig. pub. 1978.)

———. 1985. *The use of pleasure.* Vol. 2 of *The history of sexuality.* Trans. R. Hurley. New York: Random House. (Orig. pub. 1976.)

———. 1986. *The care of the self.* Vol. 3 of *The history of sexuality.* Trans. R. Hurley. New York: Random House. (Orig. pub. 1976.)

———. 1991. "Governmentality." In Burchell, Gordon, and Miller 1991, 87–104.

Fox, N. J. 1992. *The social meaning of surgery.* Milton Keynes, U.K.: Open Univ. Press.

Fox, R. 1957. "Training for uncertainty." In *The student-physician,* eds. R. K. Merton, G. Reader, and P. L. Kendall. Cambridge, Mass.: Harvard Univ. Press.

Fox, R. 2000. "Medical uncertainty revisited." In Albrecht, Fitzpatrick, and Scrimshaw 2000, 409–25.

Frank, G. 1984. "Life history model of adaptation to disability: The case of a 'congenital amputee.' " *Social Science & Medicine* 19 (6): 639–45.

———. 1986. "On embodiment: A case of congenital limb deficiency in American culture." *Culture, Medicine & Psychiatry* 10:189–219.

Frank, A. W. 1990. "Bringing bodies back in: A decade review." *Theory, Culture & Society* 7:131–62.

———. 1991a. *At the will of the body: Reflections on illness.* Boston: Houghton Mifflin.

———. 1991b. "From sick role to health role: Deconstructing Parsons." In *Talcott Parsons: Theorist of modernity,* ed. R. Robertson and B. S. Turner, 205–16. London: SAGE.

———. 1995. *The wounded storyteller: Body, illness, and ethics.* Chicago: Univ. of Chicago Press.

———. 2000. "Illness and the interactionist vocation." *Symbolic Interaction* 23 (4): 321–32.

———. 2001. "Can we research suffering?" *Qualitative Health Research* 11 (3): 353–62.

Freidan, B. 1993. *The fountain of age.* New York: Simon & Schuster.

Friedman, M., and R. H. Rosenman. 1959. "Association of specific overt behavior pattern with blood and cardiovascular findings." *Journal of the American Medical Association* 169:1286–96.

Friedson, E. 1970. *Profession of medicine: A study of the sociology of applied knowledge.* New York: Harper & Row.

Fryer, G. E., Jr. 1991. "The United States medical profession: An abnormal form of the division of labour." *Sociology of Health & Illness* 13 (2): 213–30.

Fujiura, G. T., and V. Rutkowski-Kmitta. 2001. "Counting disability." In Albrecht, Seelman, and Bury 1991, 69–96.

Fukuyama, F. 2002. *Our posthuman future: Consequences of the biotechnology revolution.* New York: Farrar, Straus & Giroux.

Gadamer, H.-G. 1996. *The enigma of health: The art of healing in a scientific age.* Trans. J. Gaiger and N. Walker. Cambridge: Polity Press.

Galea, S., A. Karpati, and B. Kennedy. 2002. "Social capital and violence in the United States: 1974–1993." *Social Science & Medicine* 55 (8): 1373–84.

Gane, M. 2003. *French social theory.* London: SAGE.

Garrett, C. J. 1996. "Recovery from anorexia nervosa: A Durkheimian interpretation." *Social Science & Medicine* 43 (10): 1489–1506.

Garrett, I. 1995. *The coming plague: Newly emerging diseases in a world out of balance.* London: Virago.

Gehlen, A. 1980. *Man in the age of technology.* New York: Columbia Univ. Press.

———. 1988. *Man: His nature and place in the world.* New York: Columbia Univ. Press.

Gerhardt, U. 1987. "Parsons, role theory, and health interaction." In *Sociological theory and medical sociology,* 110–33. London: Tavistock.

———. 1989. *Ideas about illness: An intellectual and political history of medical sociology.* London: Macmillan.

Giddens, A. 1990. *The consequences of modernity.* Cambridge: Polity Press.

———. 1991. *Modernity and self-identity: Self and society in the late modern age.* Cambridge: Polity Press.

———. 1992. *The transformation of intimacy: Sexuality, love, and eroticism in modern societies.* Cambridge: Polity Press.

Giffin, K., and C. M. Lowndes. 1999. "Gender, sexuality, and the prevention of sexually transmissible diseases." *Social Science & Medicine* 48 (3): 283–92.

Glaser, B. G., and A. L. Strauss. 1965. *Awareness of dying.* Chicago: Aldine.

———. 1968a. *Time for dying.* Chicago: Aldine.

———. 1968b. *The discovery of grounded theory: Strategies for qualitative research.* London: Weidenfeld & Nicolson.

———. 1970. *Anguish: The case history of a dying trajectory.* Mill Valley, Calif.: Sociology Press.

———. 1971. *Status passage: A formal theory.* Chicago: Aldine.

Goffman, E. 1961. *Asylums: Essays on the social situation of mental patients and other inmates.* Harmondsworth, U.K.: Penguin.

———. 1964. *Stigma: Notes on the management of spoiled identity.* Englewood Cliffs, N.J.: Prentice Hall.

Gott, M., and S. Hinchliff. 2003. "How important is sex in later life? The view of older people." *Social Science & Medicine* 56 (8): 1617–28.

Gove, W. R., and M. R. Geerken. 1977. "The Effect of Children and Employment on the Mental Health of Married Men and Women." *Social Forces* 56:66–77.

Graham, H. 1984. *Women, health, and the family*. Brighton, U.K.: Wheatsheaf.

Gravelle, H. 1998. "How much of the relationship between population morality and unequal distribution of income is a statistical artefact?" *British Medical Journal* 316:382–85.

Green, B. S. 1993. *Gerontology and the construction of old age: A study in discourse analysis*. New York: Aldine de Gruyter.

Green, A., S. Day, and H. Ward. 2000. "Crack cocaine and prostitution in London in the 1990s." *Sociology of Health & Illness* 22 (1): 27–39.

Guerrini, A. 1989. "Isaac Newton, George Cheyne, and the 'Principia medicinae.' " In *The medical revolution of the seventeenth century*, ed. R. French and A. Weir, 222–45. Cambridge: Cambridge Univ. Press.

Habermas, J. 1976. *Legitimation crisis*. London: Heinemann.

Hacking, I. 1999. *The social construction of what?* Cambridge: Harvard Univ. Press.

Hallam, E., J. Hockey, and G. Howarth. 1999. *Beyond the body: Death and social identity*. London: Routledge.

Hansen, E. C., 2001. "Medical understandings of lifestyle: An interpretive study of 'life-style' as a medical explanatory framework." PhD diss., Univ. of Tasmania, Australia.

Haraway, D. 1991. *Symians, cyborgs, and women: The reinvention of nature*. London: Free Association Books.

Hawe, P., and A. Shiell. 2000. "Social capital and health promotion: A review." *Social Science & Medicine* 51 (6): 871–85.

Hayek, F. A. 1944. *The road to serfdom*. London: Routledge.

Heggenhougen, H. K. 2000. "More than just 'interesting!' Anthropology, health, and human rights." *Social Science & Medicine* 50 (9): 1171–75.

Heidegger, M. 1958. *The question of being*. Trans. W. Klubach and J. T. Wilde. New York: Twayne.

Held, D. 1995. *Democracy and the global order: From the modern state to cosmopolitan governance*. Cambridge: Polity Press.

Held, D., A. McGrew, D. Goldblatt, and J. Perraton. 1999. *Global transformations: Politics, economics, and culture*. Cambridge: Polity Press.

Hepworth, M. 2000. *Stories of ageing*. Buckingham, U.K.: Open Univ. Press.

Hertzman, C. 2000. "Social change, market forces, and health." *Social Science & Medicine* 51 (7): 1007–8.

Hertzman, C., and A. Siddiqi. 2000. "Health and rapid economic change in the late twentieth century." *Social Science & Medicine* 51 (6): 809–19.

Higgins, P. 1980. *Outsiders in a hearing world: A sociology of deafness*. Beverly Hills, Calif.: SAGE.

Higgs, H., ed. 1931. *Richard Cantillon: Essay on the nature of commerce in general*. London: Royal Economics Society.

Hirst, P., and G. Thompson. 1996. *Globalization in question*. Cambridge: Polity Press.

Hitchcock, T. 1997. *English sexualities: 1700–1800*. London: Macmillan.

Hocking, J., and A. James. 1993. *Growing up and growing old: Ageing and dependency in the life course*. London: SAGE.

Hughes, B., and K. Paterson. 1997. "The social model of disability and the disappearing body: Towards a sociology of impairment." *Disability & Society* 12 (3): 325–40.

Huntington, S. 1997. *The clash of civilisations and the remaking of the world*. New York: Simon & Schuster.

Hutton, W. 2000. *New life for health*. London: Vintage.

Hyden, L.-C. 1997. "Illness and narrative." *Sociology of Health & Illness* 19 (1): 48–69.

Illich, I. 1977. *The limits of medicine, medical nemesis: The expropriation of health*. Harmondsworth, U.K.: Penguin.

Illouz, E. 1997. *Consuming the Romantic utopia: Love and the cultural contradictions of capitalism*. Berkeley: Univ. of California Press.

Ingstad, B., and S. R. Whyte, eds. 1995. *Disability and culture*. Berkeley: Univ. of California Press.

Jenkins, P. 1994. *Using murder: The social construction of the serial killer*. New York: Aldine de Gruyter.

Jette, A. M. 1999. "Disentangling the process of disablement." *Social Science & Medicine* 48 (4): 471–72.

Jones, C., and R. Porter, eds. 1994. *Reassessing Foucault: Power, medicine, and the body*. London: Routledge.

Jordanova, L. 1995. "The social construction of medical knowledge." *Social History of Medicine* 8 (3): 361–81.

Kalb, D., M. van der Land, R. Staring, B. van Steenbergen, and N. Wilterdink, eds. 2000. *The ends of globalization: Bringing society back in*. Lanham, Md.: Rowman & Littlefield.

Kalucy, R. S., A. H. Crisp, and B. Harding. 1977. "A study of 56 families with anorexia nervosa." *British Journal of Medical Psychology* 50:381–95.

Kaplan, G. A., E. Pamuk, J. W. Lynch, R. D. Cohen, and J. L. Balfour. 1996. "Income inequality and mortality in the United States: Analysis of mortality and potential pathways." *British Medical Journal* 312:999–1003.

Kass, L. R. 2002. *Life, liberty, and the defense of dignity: The challenge for bioethics*. San Francisco: Encounter Books.

Katz, S. 1996. *Disciplining old age: The formation of gerontological knowledge*. Charlottesville: Univ. of Virginia Press.

Kawachi, I., and B. P. Kennedy. 1997. "Health and social cohesion: Why care about income inequality?" *British Medical Journal* 314:1037–40.

———. 2002. *The health of nations: Why inequality is harmful to your health.* New York: New Press.

Kawachi, I., B. P. Kennedy, V. Gupta, and D. Preothrow-Stith. 1999. "Women's status and the health of women and men: A view from the States." *Social Science & Medicine* 48 (1): 21–32.

Kawachi, I., B. P. Kennedy, and R. G. Wilkinson. 1999. "Crime: Social disorganisation and relative deprivation." *Social Science & Medicine* 48 (6): 719–31.

Kemeny, J. 1984. "The social construction of housing facts." *Scandinavian Housing & Planning Research* 1:149–64.

King, L. S. 1982. *Medical thinking: A historical preface.* Princeton, N.J.: Princeton Univ. Press.

Kirkland, G. 1986. *Dancing on my grave: An autobiography.* With G. Lawrence. Garden City, N.Y.: Doubleday.

Kleinman, A. 1988. *The illness narratives: Suffering, healing, and the human condition.* New York: Basic Books.

Kleinman, A., V. Das, and M. Lock, eds. 1997. *Social suffering.* Berkeley: Univ. of California Press.

Kleinman, A., and J. Kleinman, eds. 1996. "Social suffering." Special issue, *Daedalus* 125 (1): 1–24.

Klinenberg, E. 2002. *Heat wave: A social autopsy of disaster in Chicago.* Chicago: Univ. of Chicago Press.

Kramer, P. D. 1994. *Listening to Prozac.* London: Fourth Estate.

Krieger, N., D. L. Rowley, A. A. Herman, B. Avery, and M. T. Phillips. 1993. "Racism, sexism, and social class: Implications for studies of health, disease, and well-being." *American Journal of Preventive Medicine* 9 (6): S82–S122.

Kroker, A., and M. Kroker, eds. 1987. *Body invaders: Panic sex in America.* New York: St. Martin's Press.

Kubisch, A. C., and R. Stone. 2001. "Comprehensive community initiatives: The American experience." In *Rebuilding community: Policy and practice in urban regeneration*, ed. J. Pierson and J. Smith, 13–33. Basingstoke, U.K.: Palgrave.

Kuh, D., R. Hardy, B. Rodgers, and M. E. J. Wadsworth. 2002. "Lifetime risk factors for women's psychological distress in midlife." *Social Science & Medicine* 55 (11): 1957–74.

Laqueur, T. 1990. *Making sex: Body and gender from the Greeks to Freud.* Cambridge, Mass.: Harvard Univ. Press.

Larson, M. S. 1977. *The rise of professionalism: A sociological analysis.* Berkeley: Univ. of California Press.

Lash, S., B. Szerszynski, and B. Wynne, eds. 1996. *Risk, environment, and modernity: Towards a new ecology.* London: SAGE.

Lasker, J. N., B. P. Egolf, and S. Wolf. 1994. "Community, social change, and mortality." *Social Science & Medicine* 39 (3): 53–62.

Latkin, C. A., and A. D. Curry. 2003. "Stressful neighborhoods and depression: A prospective study of the impact of neighborhood disorder." *Journal of Health & Social Behavior* 44 (1): 34–44.

Lehoux, P., C. Sicotte, J.-L. Denis, M. Berg, and A. Lacroix. 2002. "The theory of use behind telemedicine: How compatible with physicians' clinical routines." *Social Science & Medicine* 54 (6): 669–904.

Lewins, F. 1995. *Transsexualism in Society: A sociology of male-to-female transsexuals.* Melbourne: Macmillan.

Light, D. W. 2001. "Comparative institutional response to economic policy, managed competition, and governmentality." *Social Science & Medicine* 52 (8): 1151–66.

Lin, N. 2001. *Social capital: A theory of social structure and action.* Cambridge: Cambridge Univ. Press.

Lock, M. 1993. *Encounters with aging: Mythologies of menopause in Japan and North America.* Berkeley: Univ. of California Press.

Lock, M., A. Young, and A. Cambrosio, eds. 2000. *Living and working with the new medical technologies: Intersections of inquiry.* Cambridge: Cambridge Univ. Press.

Lomas, J. 1998. "Social capital and health: Implications for public health and epidemiology." *Social Science & Medicine* 47 (9): 1181–88.

Lorber, J., and L. J. Moore. 2002. *Gender and the social construction of illness.* Lanham, Md.: Rowman & Littlefield.

Love, J. 2003. "Prescription for pain." *Le monde diplomatique* (March): 15.

Lynch, J. J. 1977. *The broken heart: The medical consequences of loneliness.* Cambridge: Basic Books.

Lynch, J. W. 2000. "Income inequality and health: Expanding the debate." *Social Science & Medicine* 51 (7): 1001–5.

Lyons, A. C., and C. Griffin. 2003. "Managing menopause: A qualitative analysis of self-help literature for women at midlife." *Social Science & Medicine* 56 (8): 1629–42.

Lyotard, J.-F. 1984. *The postmodern condition: A report on knowledge.* Trans. G. Bennington and B. Massumi. Minneapolis: Univ. of Minnesota Press.

Macintyre, S. 1997. "The Black Report and beyond: What are the issues?" *Social Science & Medicine* 44 (6): 723–45.

Maddi, S. R., and S. C. Kobasa. 1984. *The hardy executive: Health under stress.* Homewood, Ill.: Dow Jones–Irwin.

Mamo, L., and J. R. Fishman. 2001. "Potency in all the right places: Viagra as a technology of the gendered body." *Body & Society* 7 (4): 13–35.

Mann, J., L. Goston, S. Gruskin, R. Brennan, Z. Lazzarini, and H. Fineberg. 1994. "Health and human rights." *Health & Human Rights* 1 (1): 6–23.

Marmot, M. G., and G. Davey Smith. 1997. "Socio-economic differentials in health." *Journal of Health Psychology* 2 (3): 283–96.

Marshall, T. H. 1963. *Sociology at the cross roads.* London: Heinemann.

Martin, E. 1987. *The woman in the body: A cultural analysis of reproduction.* Milton Keynes, U.K.: Open Univ. Press.

Martin, L. H., H. Gutman, and P. H. Hutton, eds. 1988. *Technologies of the self.* London: Tavistock.

Marx, K. 1964. *The economic and philosophical manuscripts.* New York: International.

Masse, R., and F. Legare. 2001. "The limitations of a negotiation model for perimenopausal women." *Sociology of Health & Illness* 23 (1): 44–64.

May, C., and D. Sirur. 1998. "Art, science, and placebo: Incorporating homeopathy in general practice." *Sociology of Health & Illness* 20 (2): 168–90.

Maynard, D. W. 1991. "Interaction and asymmetry in clinical discourse." *American Journal of Sociology* 97 (2): 448–95.

McDonnell, O. 2001. "New reproductive technologies and public discourse: From biopolitics to bioethics." PhD diss., National Univ. of Ireland, Cork.

McDonough, P., and V. Walters. 2001. "Gender and health: Reassessing patterns and explanations." *Social Science & Medicine* 52 (4): 547–59.

McKeown, T. 1979. *The role of medicine: Dream, mirage, or nemesis?* Oxford: Basil Blackwell.

McKinlay, J. B., and J. Stoeckle. 1988. "Corporatization and social transformation of doctoring." *International Journal of Health Services* 18 (2): 191–205.

McKinlay, J. B., and L. D. Marceau. 1998. "The impact of managed care on patients' trust in medical care and their physicians." Paper presented at the meeting of the American Public Health Association, Washington, D.C. Cited in Cockerham 2001, 196.

McLuhan, M. 1960. *Explorations in communication.* Boston: Beacon Press.

———. 1962. *The Gutenberg galaxy: The making of typographic man.* London: Routledge & Kegan Paul.

McNeill, W. H. 1976. *Plagues and peoples.* Oxford: Basil Blackwell.

Mead, M. 1935. *Sex and temperament in three primitive societies.* New York: W. Morrow.

Milio, N. 1985. "US public policies make you sick." *Radical Community Medicine,* 25–34.

Mills, C. W. 1956. *The power elite.* New York: Simon & Schuster.

———. 1959. *The sociological imagination.* Oxford: Oxford Univ. Press.

Mirowsky, J. 1995. "Age and the sense of control." *Social Psychology Quarterly* 58:31–43.

Mitchell, D. T., and S. L. Snyder, eds. 1997. *The body and physical difference: Discourses of disability.* Ann Arbor: Univ. of Michigan Press.

Mitchell, J. 2000. *Mad men and Medusas: Reclaiming hysteria and the effect of sibling relationships on the human condition.* London: Allen Lane.

Moore, B. 1970. *Reflections on the causes of human misery and upon certain proposals to eliminate them.* Boston: Beacon Press.

Moore, W. E. 1966. "Global sociology: The world as a singular system." *American Journal of Sociology* 71 (5): 475–82.

Moran, M. 1999. *Governing the health care state: A comparative study of the United Kingdom, the United States, and Germany.* Manchester, U.K.: Manchester Univ. Press.

Mulkay, M. 1997. *The embryo research debate: Science and the politics of reproduction.* Cambridge: Cambridge Univ. Press.

Mulkay, M., and J. Ernst. 1991. "The changing profile of social death." *European Journal of Sociology* 32 (4): 172–96.

Mumford, E. 1983. *Medical sociology, patients providers, and policies.* New York: London House.

Musick, M., and J. Wilson. 2003. "Volunteering and depression: The role of psychological and social resources in different age groups." *Social Science & Medicine* 56 (2): 259–69.

Nagi, S. 1976. "An epidemiology of disability among adults in the United States." *Milbank Quarterly* 54:439–67.

Navarro, V. 1976. *Medicine under capitalism.* New York: Prodist.

———. 1986. *Crisis, health, and medicine: A social critique.* New York: Tavistock.

Navarro, V., and D. M. Berman, eds. 1977. *Health and work under capitalism: An international perspective.* Farmingdale, N.Y.: Baywood.

Nederveen Pieterse, J. 1995. "Globalization as hybridization." In Featherstone, Lash, and Robertson. 45–68.

Newby, H. 1996. "Citizenship in a green world: Global commons and human stewardship." In *Citizenship today: The contemporary relevance of T. H. Marshall.* ed. M. Bulmer and A. M. Rees, 209–22. London: UCL Press.

Niezen, R. 2000. *Spirit wars: Native North American religions in the age of nation building.* Berkeley: Univ. of California Press.

Nigenda, G., L. Lockett, C. Monca, and G. Mora. 2001. "Non-biomedical health care practices in the state of Morelos, Mexico: Analysis of an emergent phenomenon. *Sociology of Health & Illness* 23 (1): 3–23.

Northouse, P., and L. Northouse. 1987. "Communication and cancer: Issues confronting patients, health professionals, and family members." *Journal of Psychosocial Oncology* 5 (3): 17–46.

Nussbaum, M. C. 2000. *Women and human development: The capabilities approach.* Cambridge: Cambridge Univ. Press.

Oberg, P. 1996. "The Absent Body—A social gerontological paradox." *Ageing & Society* 16:701–19.

Offer, A. 2001. "Body weight and self-control in the United States and Britain since the 1950s." *Social History of Medicine* 14 (1): 79–106.

O'Neill, J. 1990. "AIDS as a globalising panic." *Theory, Culture & Society* 7 (2–3): 329–42.

Ong, A. 1999. *Flexible citizenship: The cultural logics of transnationality.* Durham, N.C.: Duke University Press.

Orbach, S. 1978. *Fat is a feminist issue.* New York: Paddington Press.

Orona, C. J. 1990. "Temporality and identity loss due to Alzheimer's disease." *Social Science & Medicine* 30 (11): 1247–56.

Palmer, R. L. 1979. "The dietary chaos syndrome: A useful new term." *British Journal of Medical Psychology* 52:187–90.

———. 1980. *Anorexia nervosa.* Harmondsworth, U.K.: Penguin.

Parlee, M. B. 1994. "The social construction of premenstrual syndrome: A case study of scientific discourse as cultural contestation." In *The good body: Asceticism in contemporary culture,* ed. M. G. Winkler and L. B. Cole, 91–107. New Haven, Conn.: Yale Univ. Press.

Parmenter, T. R. 2001. "Disability and the sociology of the body." In Albrecht, Seelman, and Scrimshaw 2001, 252–66.

Parsons, T. 1937. *The structure of social action.* New York: McGraw-Hill.

———. 1951. *The social system.* London: Routledge & Kegan Paul.

———. "Illness and the role of the physician: A sociological perspective." In Turner 1999c, 101–8.

———. 1999b. "Youth in the context of American society." In Turner 1999c, 271–91.

Pateman, C., and E. Gross, eds. 1986. *Feminist challenges: Social and political theory.* Sydney: George Allen & Unwin.

Patton, C. 1990. *Inventing AIDS.* New York: Routledge.

Pescosolido, B. A., and C. A. Boyer. 2001. "The American health care system: Entering the twenty-first century with high risk, major challenges, and great opportunities." In Cockerham 2001, 180–98.

Petersen, A., and R. Bunton, eds. 1997. *Foucault, health, and medicine.* London: Routledge.

Petersen, A., and D. Lupton. 1996. *The new public health: Health and self in an age of risk.* St. Leonards, Australia: George Allen & Unwin.

Phillipson, C. 1998. *Reconstructing old age: New agendas in social theory and practice.* London: SAGE.

Pickering, W. S. F., ed. 2002. *Durkheim today.* London: Routledge.

Pierret, J. 2003. "The illness experience—State of knowledge and perspectives for research." *Sociology of Health & Illness* 25 (1): 4–22.

Pitts, V. 2003. *In the flesh: The cultural politics of body modification.* Basingstoke, U.K.: Palgrave.

Plummer, K. 2000. "Symbolic interactionism in the twentieth century." In Turner 2000d, 193–222.

Porter, D., ed. 1997. *Social medicine and medical sociology in the twentieth century.* Atlanta: Editions Rodopi B. V. Amsterdam.

Porter, R. 1997. *The greatest benefit to mankind: A medical history of humanity from antiquity to the present.* London: HarperCollins.

———. 2001. *Bodies politic: Disease, death, and doctors in Britain, 1650–1900.* London: Reaktion Books.

Portes, A. 1998. "Social capital: Its origins and applications in modern sociology." *Annual Review of Sociology* 24:1–24.

Putnam, R. D. 1993. *Making democracy work: Civic traditions in modern Italy.* With R. Leonardi and R. Y. Nanetti. Princeton, N.J.: Princeton Univ. Press.

———. 2000. *Bowling alone: The collapse and revival of American community.* New York: Touchstone.

Radley, A. 1999. "The aesthetics of illness: Narrative, horror, and the sublime." *Sociology of Health & Illness* 21 (6): 778–96.

Rawls, J. 1970. *A theory of justice.* Oxford: Oxford Univ. Press.

Redden, C. J. 2002. *Health care, entitlement, and citizenship.* Toronto: Univ. of Toronto Press.

Rhodes, T., and L. Cusick. 2000. "Love and intimacy in relationship risk management: HIV positive people and their sexual partners." *Sociology of Health & Illness* 22 (1): 1–26.

Richards, M. P. M. 1993. "The new genetics: Some issues for social scientists." *Sociology of Health & Illness* 15 (5): 567–86.

Richardson, D. 2000. *Rethinking sexuality.* London: SAGE.

Richardson, D., and S. Seidman, eds. 2002. *Handbook of lesbian and gay studies.* London: SAGE.

Rietschlin, J. 1998. "Voluntary association membership and psychological distress." *Journal of Health & Social Behavior* 39 (4): 348–55.

Riggs, A., and B. S. Turner. 1999. "The expectation of love in older age: Towards a sociology of intimacy." In *A certain age: Women growing older,* ed. M. Poole and S. Feldman, 193–208. St. Leonards: George Allen & Unwin.

Rinken, S. 2000. *The AIDS crisis and the modern self: Biographical self-construction in the awareness of finitude.* Boston: Kluwer.

Riska, E. 2002. "From type A man to the hardy man: Masculinity and health." *Sociology of Health & Illness* 24 (3): 347–58.

Ritzer, G. 2000. *The McDonaldization of society.* Thousand Oaks, Calif.: Pine Forge Press.

Robert, S. A., and J. S. House. 2000. "Socioeconomic inequalities in health: Integrating individual-, community- and societal-level theory and research." In Albrecht, Fitzpatrick, and Scrimshaw 2000, 115–35.

Robertson, R. 1992. *Globalization: Social theory and global culture.* London: SAGE.

Rock, M. 2000. "Discounted lives? Weighing disability when measuring health and ruling on 'compassionate' murder." *Social Science & Medicine* 51 (3): 407–17.

Rogers, M. S. 1999. "Pain talk in oncology outpatient clinics." PhD diss., University of Cambridge, Cambridge.

Rojek, C., and B. S. Turner. 2000. "Decorative sociology." *Sociological Review* 48 (4): 629–48.

Rorty, R. 1989. *Contingency, Irony, and Solidarity.* Cambridge: Cambridge Univ. Press.

———. 1998. *Truth and Progress.* Cambridge: Cambridge Univ. Press.

Rose, N. 1989. *Governing the soul: The shaping of the private self.* London: Routledge.

Roth, J. A. 1963. *Timetables.* Indianapolis, Ind.: Bobbs-Merrill.

———. 1984. "Staff-inmate bargaining tactics in long-term treatment institutions." *Sociology of Health & Illness* 6 (2): 111–31.

Roth, J. A., and P. Conrad, eds. 1987. *The experience and management of chronic illness.* Greenwich, Conn.: JAI Press.

Rothman, B. K. 1998. *Genetic maps and human imaginations: The limits of science in understanding who we are.* New York: W. W. Norton.

Rothstein, W. G. 1987. *American medical schools and the practice of medicine: A history.* Oxford: Oxford Univ. Press.

Rousselle, A. 1988. *Porneia: On desire and the body in antiquity.* Trans. F. Pheasant. Oxford: Basil Blackwell.

Sacks, O. 1976. *Awakenings.* Harmondsworth, U.K.: Penguin.

———. 1985. *The man who mistook his wife for a hat.* London: Gerald Duckworth.

———. 1989. *Seeing voices: A journey into the world of the deaf.* Berkeley and Los Angeles: Univ. of California Press.

Salander, P. 2002. "Bad news from the patient's perspective: An analysis of the written narratives of newly diagnosed cancer patients." *Social Science & Medicine* 55 (5): 721–32.

Samson, C., ed. 1999. *Health studies: A critical and cross-cultural reader.* Oxford: Basil Blackwell.

Sassen, S. 1999. *Guests and aliens.* New York: New Press.

Scheper-Hughes, N. 1992. *Death without weeping: The violence of everyday life in Brazil.* Berkeley: Univ. of California Press.

———. 2001a. "Neo-cannibalism: The global trade in human organs." *Hedgehog Review* 3 (2): 7–52.

———. 2001b. "Commodity fetishism in organs trafficking." *Body & Society* 7 (2–3): 31–62.

Schieman, S., and H. A. Turner. 1998. "Age, disability, and the sense of mastery." *Journal of Health & Social Behavior* 39 (3): 169–86.

Schudson, M. 1998. *The good citizen: A history of American civil life.* New York: Free Press.

Scott, A. 1998. "Homeopathy as a feminist form of medicine." *Sociology of Health & Illness* 20 (2): 191–215.

Scott, A. J. 2000. *The cultural economy of cities.* London: SAGE.

Scully, D., and P. Bart. 1978. "A funny thing happened on the way to the orifice: Women in gynecology textbooks." In *The cultural crisis of modern medicine,* ed. J. Ehrenreich. New York: Monthly Review Press.

Sen, A. 1999. *Development as freedom.* Oxford: Oxford Univ. Press.

Sennett, R. 1998. *The corrosion of character: The personal consequences of work in the new capitalism.* New York: W. W. Norton.

———. 2003. *Respect: The formation of character in an age of inequality.* London: Allen Lane.

Seymour, W. 1989. *Bodily alterations: An introduction to a sociology of the body for health work-ers.* Sydney: George Allen & Unwin.

———. 1998. *Remaking the body: Rehabilitation and change.* St. Leonards, Australia: George Allen & Unwin.

Shakespeare, T., and N. Watson. 1995. "Defending the social model." *Disability & Society* 12 (2): 293–300.

Shilling, C. 1993. *The body and social theory.* London: SAGE.

Siegrist, J. 2000. "The social causation of health and illness." In Albrecht, Fitzpatrick, and Scrimshaw 2000, 101–14.

Sigerist, H. E. 1951. *Primitive and archaic medicine.* Vol. 1 of *A history of medicine.* Oxford: Oxford Univ. Press.

Singer, P. 1979. *Practical ethics.* Cambridge: Cambridge Univ. Press.

———. 1994. *Rethinking life and death: The collapse of our traditional ethics.* Oxford: Oxford Univ. Press.

Sjoberg, G., E. A. Gill, and N. Williams. 2001. "A sociology of human rights." *Social Prob-lems* 48 (1): 11–47.

Smart, A. 2003. "Reporting the dawn of the post-genomic era: Who wants to live forever?" *Sociology of Health & Illness* 25 (1): 50–70.

Sontag, S. 1978. *Illness as metaphor.* New York: Vintage.

———. 1989. *AIDS and its metaphors.* New York: Farrar, Straus & Giroux.

Star, S. L., and G. C. Bowker. 1997. "Of Lungs and lungers: The classified story of tuber-culosis." In Strauss and Corbin 1997, 197–227.

Starr, P. 1982. *The social transformation of American medicine: The rise of a sovereign profession and the making of a vast industry.* New York: Basic Books.

Steinbrugge, L. 1995. *The moral sex: Woman's nature in the French Enlightenment.* New York: Oxford Univ. Press.

Stevens, R. 1998. *American medicine and the public interest: A history of specialization.* Berkeley: Univ. of California Press.

Stiker, H.-J. 1982. *Corps infirmes et societes.* Paris: Aubier Montaigne.

Strauss, A. L. 1959. *Mirrors and masks: The search for identity.* Glencoe, Ill.: Free Press.

Strauss, A. L., L. Schatzman, D. Ehrlich, R. Bucher, and M. Sabshin. 1963. "The hospital and its negotiated order." In *The hospital in modern society*, ed. E. Friedson. New York: Free Press of Glencoe.

———. 1978. *Negotiations: Varieties, contexts, processes, and social order.* San Francisco: Jossey-Bass.

———. 1993. *Continual permutations of action.* New York: Aldine de Gruyter.

Strauss, A. L., and J. Corbin, eds. 1997. *Grounded theory in practice.* Thousand Oaks, Calif.: SAGE.

Strauss, A. L., S. Fagerhaugh, B. Suczek, and C. Wiener. 1985. *Social organization of medical work.* Chicago: Univ. of Chicago Press.

Strauss, A. L., and B. Glaser. 1975. *Chronic illness and the quality of life.* St. Louis, Mo.: C. V. Mosby.

Sudnow, D. 1967. *Passing on: The social organization of dying.* Englewood Cliffs, N.J.: Prentice Hall.

Synnott, A. 1993. *The body social: Symbolism, self, and society.* London: Routledge.

Szasz, T. 1961. *The myth of mental illness.* London: Paladin.

———. 1970. *The manufacture of madness.* New York: Harper & Row.

Szreter, S. 1988. "The importance of social intervention in Britain's mortality decline, c. 1850–1914: A reinterpretation of the role of public health." *Social History of Medicine* 1 (1): 1–37.

Tarlov, A. R. 2000. "Coburn's thesis: Plausible, but we need more evidence and better measures." *Social Science & Medicine* 51 (7): 993–96.

Taylor, R., and A. Rieger. 1984. "Rudolf Virchow on the typhus epidemic in Upper Silesia." *Sociology of Health & Illness* 6 (2): 201–17.

Thoits, P. A., and L. N. Hewitt. 2001. "Volunteer work and well-being." *Journal of Health & Social Behavior* 42 (2): 115–31.

Thomas, C. 2002. "The 'Disabled' Body." In *Real bodies: A sociological introduction,* ed. M. Evans and E. Lee, 64–78. Houndmills, U.K.: Palgrave.

Titmuss, R. M. 1970. *The gift relationship: From human blood to social policy.* London: George Allen & Unwin.

Tocqueville, A. de 1959. *Journey to America.* Trans. G. Lawrence. New Haven, Conn.: Yale Univ. Press.

———. 1968. *Democracy in America.* Glasgow: Collins. (Orig. pub. 1835–40.)

Toombs, K. S. 1995. "The lived experience of disability." *Human studies* 18:9–23.

Tourraine, A. 2000. *Can we live together? Equality and difference.* Cambridge: Polity Press.

Townsend, P., and N. Davidson. 1982. *Inequalities in health.* Harmondsworth, U.K.: Pelican Books.

Trieber, F., T. Batanowski, D. Broden, W. Strong, M. Levy, and W. Knox. 1991. "Social support for exercise: Relationship to physical activity in young adults." *Preventive Medicine* 20:737–50.

Turner, B. S. 1981. *For Weber: Essays on the sociology of fate.* London: Routledge & Kegan Paul.

———. 1982. "The government of the body: Medical regimens and the rationalization of diet." *British Journal of Sociology* 33 (2): 254–69.

———. 1984. *The body and society: Explorations in social theory.* Oxford: Basil Blackwell.

———. 1992. *Regulating bodies: Essays in medical sociology.* London: Routledge.

———, ed. 1993. *Citizenship and social theory.* London: SAGE.

———. 1994a. "Postmodern culture/modern citizens." In *The condition of citizenship,* ed. B. van Steinberg, 153–68. London: SAGE.

———. 1994b. "The postmodernisation of the life course: Towards a new social gerontology." *Australian Journal on Ageing* 13 (3): 109–11.

———. 1995a. *Medical power and social knowledge.* London: SAGE.

———. 1995b. "Ageing and identity: Some reflections on the somatization of the self." In Featherstone and Wernick 1995, 245–60.

———. 1996. *Body & Society.* 2nd ed. London: SAGE.

———. 1997a. "A neo-Hobbesian theory of human rights: A reply to Malcolm Waters." *Sociology* 31 (3): 565–71.

———. 1997b. "What is the sociology of the body?" *Body & Society* 3 (1): 103–7.

———. 1997c. "From governmentality to risk: Some reflections on Foucault's contribution to medical sociology." In Petersen and Bunton 1997, ix–xxi.

———. 1998a. Foreword to *Remaking the body* by W. Seymour. St. Leonards, Australia: George Allen & Unwin.

———. 1998b. "Forgetfulness and frailty: Otherness and rights in contemporary social theory." In *The politics of Jean-François Lyotard: Justice and political theory,* ed. C. Rojek and B. S. Turner, 25–42. London: Routledge.

———. 1999a. "McCitizens: Risk, coolness, and irony in contemporary politics." In *Resisting McDonaldization,* ed. B. Smart, 83–100. London: SAGE.

———. 1999b. "Citizenship and health as a scarce resource." In *Second opinion: An introduction to health sociology,* ed. J. Germov, 302–14. Melbourne: Oxford Univ. Press.

———, ed. 1999c. *The Talcott Parsons reader.* Oxford: Basil Blackwell.

———. 2000a. "The history of the changing concepts of health and illness: Outline of a general model of illness categories." In Albrecht, Fitzpatrick, and Scrimshaw 2000, 9–23.

———. 2000b. "Cosmopolitan virtue: Loyalty and the city." In *Democracy, citizenship, and the global city,* ed. E. F. Isin, 129–47. London: Routledge.

———. 2000c. "Outline of a general sociology of the body." In Turner 2000d, 481–502.

———, ed. *The Blackwell companion to social theory.* Oxford: Basil Blackwell.

———. 2001a. "The end(s) of humanity." *Hedgehog Review* 3 (2): 7–32.

———. 2001b. "Risks, rights, and regulations: An overview." *Heath, Risk & Society* 3 (1): 9–18.

———. 2003a. "Social capital, inequality, and health: The Durkheimian revival." *Social Theory & Health* 1 (1): 4–20.

———. 2003b. "Social fluids: Metaphors and meanings of society." *Body & Society* 9 (1): 1–10.

Turner, B. S., and C. Rojek. 2001. *Society and culture: Principles of scarcity and solidarity.* London: SAGE.

Turner, B. S., and S. Wainwright. 2003. "Corps de ballet: The case of the injured ballet dancer." *Sociology of Health & Illness* 25 (4): 269–88.

Urry, J. 2000. "Sociology of time and space." In Turner 2000d, 416–43.

Vandenberg, A., ed. 2000. "Cybercitizenship and digital democracy." In *Citizenship and democracy in a global era,* ed. A. Vandenberg, 289–306. Basingstoke, U.K.: Macmillan.

Vaughan, M. 1991. *Curing their ills: Colonial power and African illness.* Palo Alto, Calif.: Stanford Univ. Press.

Veenstra, G. 2000. "Social capital, SES, and health: An individual-level analysis." *Social Science & Medicine* 50 (5): 619–29.

Veith, I. 1981. "Historical reflections on the changing concepts of disease." In *Concepts of health and disease: Interdisciplinary perspectives,* ed. A. L. Caplan, H. T. Engelhardt, and J. J. McCartney, 221–30. London: Addison-Wesley.

Waitzkin, H. 1983. *The second sickness: Contradictions of capitalist health care.* New York: Free Press.

Waitzkin, H., and B. Waterman. 1974. *The exploitation of illness in capitalist society.* Indianapolis, Ind.: Bobbs-Merrill.

Waldron, I. 1991. "Patterns and causes of gender differences in smoking." *Social Science & Medicine* 32 (9): 989–1005.

———. 2000. "Trends in gender differences in mortality: Relationships to changing gender differences in behaviour and other causal factors." In Annandale and Hunt 2000, 150–81.

Waldron, I., and D. Lye. 1989. "Family roles and smoking." *American Journal of Preventive Medicine* 5 (3): 136–41.

Warnock, M. 1985. *A Question of life: The Warnock report on human fertilization and embryology.* Oxford: Basil Blackwell.

———. 2002. *Making babies: Is there a right to have a child?* Oxford: Oxford Univ. Press.

Weber, M. 1930. *The Protestant ethic and the spirit of capitalism.* London: George Allen & Unwin.

Weindling, P. 1989. *Health, race, and German politics between national unification and Nazism: 1870–1945.* Cambridge: Cambridge Univ. Press.

Wernick, A. 2001. *Auguste Comte and the religion of humanity: The post-theistic program of French social theory.* Cambridge: Cambridge Univ. Press.

Whitehead, M. 1988. *The health divide.* Harmondsworth, U.K.: Penguin.

Whyte, S. R. 1995. "Disability between discourse and experience." In Ingstad and Whyte 1995, 267–92.

Whyte, W. H. 1956. *The organization man.* New York: Simon & Schuster.

Wilkinson, R. G., ed. 1986. *Class and health: Research and longitudinal data.* London: Tavistock.

———. 1992. "Income distribution and life expectancy," *British Medical Journal* 304:165–68.

———. 1996. *Unhealthy societies: The afflictions of inequality.* London: Routledge.

———. 1999. "The culture of inequality." In *The society and population health reader: Income inequality and health,* ed. I. Kawachi, B. P. Kennedy, and R. G. Wilkinson, 492–98. New York: New Press.

———. 2000. "Deeper than 'neo-liberalism': A reply to David Coburn." *Social Science & Medicine* 51 (7): 997–1000.

Williams, G. 1984. "The genesis of chronic illness: Narrative reconstruction." *Sociology of Health & Illness* 6 (2): 175–200.

Williams, S. J. 1987. "Goffman, interactionism, and stigma." In *Sociological theory and medical sociology,* ed. G. Scrambler, 134–64. London: Tavistock.

———. 1999. "Is anybody there? Critical realism, chronic illness, and the disability debate." *Sociology of Health & Illness* 21 (6): 797–819.

———. 2003. *Medicine and the body.* London: SAGE.

Wolf, S., and B. B. Berle, eds. 1981. *The technological imperative in medicine.* New York: Plenum Press.

Ziegler, P. 1998. *The black death.* London: Penguin.

Zola, I. 1972. "Medicine as an institution of social control." *Sociological Review* 20 (4): 487–504.

———. 1982. *Missing pieces: A chronicle of living with a disability.* Philadelphia: Temple Univ. Press.

———. 1988. "Aging and disability: Toward a unifying agenda." *Educational Gerontology* 14: 365–87.

———. 1989. "Toward the necessary universalizing of a disability policy." *Milbank Quarterly* 67:401–8.

———. 1991. "Bringing our bodies and ourselves back in: Reflections on a past, present, and future medical sociology." *Journal of Health & Social Behavior* 32 (1): 1–16.

INDEX

Abercrombie, N., 45
aboriginal cultures, 265
   destruction of, 262–64
abortion, 210, 218
abuse of the elderly, 187
activity theory, 146–47
adverse drug reactions, 126, 280
Afghanistan, 232
Africa, spread of HIV/AIDS in, 282–83
aging and the elderly, xix, 63, 271, 300,
      303, 304
   activity theory and, 146–47
   classification of age and aging, 164
   demographic transition and "geriatric
      diseases," xxvi
   disability and, *see* disability and impair-
      ment, aging and
   disengagement theory, 146–47, 162
   fiscal crisis in health care and, 108–9,
      118
   human vulnerability and, *see* human
      vulnerability
   lobbying and, 296
   medicalization of, 112
   moral queues and ageism, 144–45
   scarcity and, xxiii–xxiv
   sexual drive, 112
   sexual satisfaction, 85
   social constructionism and, 49, 56–57,
      147
   social gerontology, 111
   social isolation and, 24, 25, 74,
      186–87
   subjective time and, 145–46
   technology and management of, 162
   women's contribution to caring for fam-
      ily members, 300
agoraphobia, 195–96, 199

agricultural production, industrialization
   of, 260, 262, 263
AIDS, *see* HIV/AIDS
AIDS and Its Metaphors (Sontag), 154
Ajrouch, K. J., 22
Alameda County, California, studies, 4, 5
Albrecht, G. L., 44, 166, 184, 304
alcoholism, 200, 218, 300
Aleinikoff, T, A., 239
Alexander, J., 275
allopathic, Western medicine, 93–94
   Flexner Report, impact of, 106–7,
      117–18
   globalization and, 239
   historical development of, 83, 88–91,
      95–130, 276–77, 286–87
   legitimacy of, 83, 90
   Newtonian philosophy and, 95, 96–97
   see also alternative and complementary
      medicine; doctor-patient relation-
      ship; doctors
alternative and complementary medicine,
      9, 83, 90–92, 117–21, 125, 130,
      276, 278, 279, 297
   globalization and, 239
   see also allopathic, Western medicine
Altman, Dennis, 129, 243
Alzheimer's disease, 111, 206
American Medical Association, 118, 121,
      253, 277
American Sign Language (ASL), 180–82
*Anatomical Exercise on the Circulation of the
      Blood* (Harvey), 97
anatomy, 97–98, 130
Anatomy Lesson of Dr. Nicolaas Tulp, The,
      98
Anderson Cancer Center, M. D., 119
Anguish (Glaser and Strauss), 137

Full Employment in a Free Society (Beveridge), 308

Gabe, J., 249
Gadamer, Hans-Georg, 48
Galea, S., 7
Galen, 98
Gall, Franz Joseph, 33
Galludet, Thomas Hopkins, 180
Gane, M., 32
Garrett, Catherine J., 197
Garrett, I., 115
gay men, *see* homosexuality and homosexuals
Geerken, R., 201
Gehlen, Arnold, 57
gender, xix, 303–4
    alcoholism and, 200
    depression and, 17
    feminism, *see* feminism and feminist writers
    men's health, 54–56, 112, 305
    mental health and, 17, 200, 303
    sex of children, selecting the, 122, 205
    smoking and, 200–1
    sociology of the body and, 51–57
    see also sexuality
genetically modified (GM) foods, 254–55, 259, 289, 290
genetic engineering, 65, 127, 227, 280
genetic research, 206–7, 271
    regulation of, 252–56, 285
genetics, health and illness explained by, 94, 305
genetic screening, 273
Gerhardt, U., 184, 301
Germany, xvii
germ theory of disease, 103–4, 119, 296
gerontology, 165
    social, 111
Gerontology and the Construction of Old Age (Green), 164
Ghaill, M. Mac an, 238
Ghost Dance movement, 263
Giddens, A., 123, 159, 174, 177, 186, 220, 237
Giffin, K., 243
Gill, E. A., 293
Glaser, Barney G., 131, 133–34, 137, 141, 167, 168
Glass, T., 19

global governance, 266, 293
globalization, xix, 31, 35, 230–69
    antiglobalization protests, 238
    cultural McDonaldization, 238, 266
    defense of local cultures and, 238
    development of globalization theory, 235–37
    human rights and, 240–41
    infectious disease, spread of, xx, xxvii, 113–17, 123–24, 231–32, 257–58, 270–71, 275, 298–99, 304
    medical organ market, *see* organs, marketplace for
    risk and, *see* risk, globalization and
Global Sex (Altman), 243
global warming, 259
Goffman, Erving, xxiv, 135, 141, 167, 168, 189
Gold, N., 169
Golden Cage, The (Bruch), 198
Goldstein, Kurt, 78
Goodenough Committee, 110
Gordon, C., 170
Gove, W. R., 201
governmentality, xxii, 61, 82, 212–15, 217, 220
    defined, 170
    management of disability as, 171
Graham, H., 201
Gravelle, H., 24
Great Britain, *see* Britain
Greece, ancient, 237
Green, A., 232
Green, B. S., 111
Green, Bryan S., 164
Griffin, C., 54
Gross, E., 51
grounded theory, 131–32, 133–34, 167, 168
Grounded Theory in Practice (Strauss and Corbin), 138–39
Guardian, The, 289
Guerrini, A., 96
Gull, Sir William, 38
Gutenberg Galaxy, The (McLuhan), 236
Gutman, H., 63
gynecology, 194

Habermas, J., 9
Hacking, I., 40, 46
Hahnemann, Samuel, 91

INDEX ✑ 355

technology, medical, *see* medical technology
telesurgery, 128, 230–31
television, 73
terrorism, 233, 238, 240, 259, 311
    bioterrorism, 232–33, 299
thalidomide, 115, 249, 251
Thatcher, Margaret, 267, 275, 284, 288, 300
Thoits, Peggy, 21
Thomas, C., 167, 170
Thomas, H., 303
Thompson, G., 237
time, concept of
    clock time, 132
    conclusion, 160–62
    disease and, 140–47
    doctor-patient relationship and, 131, 132, 135
    life cycle, 143–44, 146
    pharmaceutical trials and, 289–90
    self and, 132–40, 158–59
    sick role and, 140–41
    subjective time, 132, 145–46
    symbolic interactionism and, 133–407
Timetables (Roth), 135
Titmuss, R. M., xxiii
Tocqueville, Alexis de, 12, 13, 16
Toombs, K. S., 170
Tourette, Gilles de la, 157
Tourette's syndrome, 157
tourist sex industry, 241
Tourraine, A., 244
Townsend, P., 110, 302
toxic shock syndrome, 114
trajectories
    of death and dying, 136–38
    of illnesses, 139
transsexuals, 177, 192
Trieber, F., 24
trust
    income inequality and life expectancy, 22
    of medical professionals, 121, 122, 123, 126, 272–73, 274, 279–80, 280, 287–88
    social capital and, 11–12, 13
tuberculosis, 76, 101, 104, 109, 123, 218, 257, 270, 271, 275, 283
Turner, Bryan S., xiv, xix, xxi, xxii, 4, 8, 31, 43, 45, 46, 63, 64, 69, 70, 75, 77, 80, 89, 96–97, 101, 109, 141,

156, 158, 160, 166, 171, 173, 185, 186, 188, 189, 191, 215, 234, 237, 240, 258, 264, 266, 292, 293, 294, 301, 309, 311
type-A men, 55–56
typhoid, 123, 275

unemployment, 201, 279, 297
Unending Work and Care (Corbin), 139
Union of the Physically Impaired Against Segregation (UPIAS), 172
United Kingdom, *see* Britain
United Nations, 265, 311
U.S. Army, 232–33
U.S. Conference of Catholic Bishops, 206
Universal Declaration of the Rights of Man, 265, 269
University of California at Berkeley, 281–82
Urry, J., 233

vaccination, 73, 94, 101, 102
Vandenberg, A., 244
Veenstra, Gerry, 19, 25
Veith, Ilza, 75
Verbrugge, L. M., 166
Vesalius, Andreas, 90, 98
Viagra, 85–86
violence, social capital and, 7
Virchow, Rudolf, 92, 93, 234
voluntary associations, 12–13, 16, 20–21, 30–31, 277, 300, 308–9
vulnerability, human, 69–74, 185, 186, 264
    as universal, 183, 188, 189, 190, 312

Wadsworth, M. E. J., 54
Wainwright, S., 77
Waitzkin, Howard, 93, 111, 289
Waldron, I., 201
Walters, V., 201
Ward, H., 232
Warnock, M., 205, 228
Waterman, B., 111, 289
Watson, N., 173
Weber, Max, 95, 247–48, 292
weight
    affluence and, 202
    eating disorders, *see* eating disorders
    gender and, 201–3
OCR